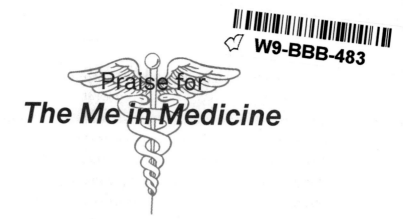
W9-BBB-483

Praise for
The Me in Medicine

"A passionate, incisive, fascinating behind-the-scenes exposé of today's flawed healthcare. *The Me in Medicine* reveals how doctors and patients have automatically bought into a 'system' that appears sound and yet disappoints. This is a must-read for doctors and patients alike—and everyone who cares about getting back to the heart of good medicine today. Sir William Osler reminded us that 'the good physician treats the disease; the great physician treats the patient who has the disease.' Likewise, the good surgeon learns how to cut; the great surgeon, like Patrick Roth, learns that the tongue may be sharper than the scalpel."

> ALAN R. COHEN, MD, Professor of Neurosurgery,
> Oncology, and Pediatrics; Chief of Pediatric Neurosurgery,
> The Johns Hopkins University School of Medicine

"Dr. Roth delivers an intriguing and entertaining review of the complicated flaws present in our current healthcare system. With compelling perspectives from history, philosophy, science and literature, Roth clarifies how we have gotten here, and where we are headed. This is a story about us, physicians and patients, and what we can do together on the ground to transform our most fundamental connections. An interesting and thought-provoking read!"

> CARL HEILMAN, MD, Chairman and Professor, Department
> of Neurosurgery, Tufts University School of Medicine

"Patrick Roth's book is important and timely. He provides incisive, real-life perspective and advice to patients and health care providers based on his decades-spanning track record as an academic neurosurgeon. He articulates what makes a physician tick. For Roth, the successful patient embarks on a journey of autonomy during which physicians and patients form a partnership. To this end, physicians must reflect on their patients' narrative. Only then can test results be placed in the clinically relevant context.

Spine surgeon Roth's bread and butter are patients with back pain whose MRIs show disk prolapses or bulges. But association does not imply causation, *post hoc non propter hoc*. As Roth explains, this misconception is the root of countless unnecessary back surgeries, poor outcomes, prolonged post-op recovery, avoidable but tremendous cost to the health care system, unimproved quality of life and dissatisfied patients. Behind this misinterpretation stands a natural but ultimately counterproductive yearning for simple explanations to complex problems—because besides disk disease, back pain is also linked to sedentary lifestyles, lack of exercise, depression and obesity, all issues for which the solutions must originate with the sufferer, not the doctor.

Roth explains persuasively what patients should seek in a good surgeon. His views rest on a keen understanding of human nature. It is not just the technical brilliance, the attention to pre- and post-op care, but also the empathy, ability and willingness to understand patients' narrative, the *sine qua non* of linking a patient's problem to the procedure and the condition for a rewarding outcome. And it is the combination of modesty and confidence that allows the doctor to admit to uncertainty and ambiguity.

I expect people who embrace Roth's thoughts and advice will become better prepared as patients and health care providers.

Florian Thomas, MD, Chair, Neurosciences,
Hackensack University Medical Center

"A thoughtful and thought-provoking book . . . regarding the critical aspects of being a physician: the patient-doctor relationship. Through this lens, Dr. Roth explores the richness and power of this relationship. . . . A beautifully written book. . . . Health professionals and patients alike will learn so much."

BONITA STANTON, MD, Dean and Professor of Pediatrics,
Seton Hall-Hackensack Meridian School of Medicine

"A call to arms to reaffirm the humanity of medicine—for both doctors and patients alike. While not shying away from the high-tech innovations that advance medical science, Roth reminds us that we can't lose sight of the primary focus of medicine: compassionate healing."

DANIELLE OFRI, MD, PhD, Author of
What Patients Say, What Doctors Hear

"*The Me in Medicine* offers a rare opportunity to peer into the heart and mind of a neurosurgeon, one who uses both his humanity and his hands to treat patients. You'll finish this remarkable book more optimistic about the future of health care."

DANIEL H. PINK, author of *When* and *Drive*

THE

ᴍE

IN

MEDICINE

Reviving the Lost Art of Healing

PATRICK ROTH, M.D.

CHANGING LIVES PRESS

The information and advice contained in this book is based upon the author's research and experiences and is the opinion of the author. They are not intended as a substitute for consulting with your physician or other healthcare provider. The publisher, author and all others who may have assisted in the publication of this work are not responsible for any adverse effects or consequences resulting from the use of any of the information or suggestions presented in this book and do not accept any liability or responsibility to any person or entity with respect to any loss or damage alleged to have been caused, directly or indirectly, by the information, ideas, opinions or other content in this book.

All matters pertaining to your physical health should be supervised by a healthcare professional that can provide medical care that is tailored to meet individual needs.

Editor: Michele Matrisciani
Cover and interior design: Gary A. Rosenberg

Changing Lives Press
P.O. Box 140189
Howard Beach, NY 11414
www.changinglivespress.com

**Library of Congress Cataloging-in-Publication Data
is on file with the Library of Congress.**

ISBN-13: 978-0-99862-316-0

Copyright © 2018 by Changing Lives Press

All rights reserved. No part of this publication may be reproduced, scanned, uploaded, stored in a retrieval system, or transmitted, in any form or by any means, electronic, mechanical, photocopying, photoediting, recording, or otherwise, without the prior written permission of the publisher, Changing Lives Press.

Printed in the United States of America

10   9   8   7   6   5   4   3   2   1

Contents

PART III. The Philosophy

PART IV. The Prescription

The Heart of a Doctor

*"May I never forget that the patient
is a fellow creature in pain.
May I never consider him
merely a vessel of disease."*
—MAIMONIDES

My Wish

An ancient Indian parable speaks of a man with bare feet who wants to walk across a field of thorns and has two options: he can pave a path in the field, or he can make himself sandals. In the former case, he sets out to change what is around him, while in the latter case, he chooses to change himself. This is not a book about changing medicine as much as a book about changing ourselves.

To Vito Victor,
the epitome of character.

INTRODUCTION

Me and Medicine

*"For where there is love of man, there is also love of the art.
For some patients, though conscious that their position is
perilous, recover their health simply through their
contentment with the physician."*

—HIPPOCRATES

More than thirty years ago I went through the process of interviewing for a neurosurgical residency. This seemed, at the time, to be the biggest decision of my life. I was graduating from medical school and now could focus on my career.

One of my interviews has always stood out, not because I was enamored with the program, but because of the very nature of the interview. I had heard stories of stress interviews, where a potential employer puts intense pressure on candidates by asking them worst-case scenario questions, testing their acumen for work overload, potential legal conflict, life-and-death situations, and so on. It is the medical version of an urban legend.

The chairman of this department was of large stature, standing well over six feet. He was commanding and intimidating and seemed generally unlikable. Instantly I knew he wasn't here to make friends. I swear he wore a monocle, but thirty years have likely embellished my memory of his appearance.

Rather than ask me about myself, he opted to pose a scenario. So much for urban legends. He wanted me to imagine I was the chairman of the department and he was a resident. He, as the resident, had failed to check a chest X-ray before a patient's surgery. He also had lied and said that he had checked it. The omission had been discovered after the surgery and, fortunately, there had been no consequences to his mistake. What was I going to do as the chairman?

I suggested that lying was unacceptable and that I would tell the resident that if he lied again, it could result in his termination from the program. The Monocle then asked me if I believed that the character of the resident could be changed, implying that surely a person late into his twenties didn't have the ability to change his nature.

"Change doesn't have a fixed expiration date," I answered confidently, despite my sweaty brow. "People can learn character at any age."

The Monocle was literally in my face at this point and exclaimed, "That was *my* resident, and I fired that son-of-a-bitch ... and I'll fire you if you ever lie to me."

Needless to say, I didn't pursue the program, but the question of character and its potential for change has remained alive in me.

Medicine is a complicated field. Within medicine, I have chosen neurosurgery. And within neurosurgery, I have chosen as my subspecialty treatment of the spine. Medicine has done a poor job with the spine, and, particularly, with low back pain. In fact, it is my opinion that the treatment of back pain is currently one of the greatest embarrassments of American medicine. The technology available today to treat the spine is incredible. We can see the spine structures in great detail with MRI. We have powerful microscopes that provide clarity through magnification and lighting. We have robots that work with computers to make us more accurate. But what I propose throughout this book will show why, despite this, we have ended up spending more money only to achieve less.

I believe that the aforementioned advances in technology have paradoxically served to worsen our treatment of back pain because they provide "easy" ways to explain the back pain. What's so wrong with easy? Nothing—except when the explanations for back pain are inaccurate and counterproductive and merely ways to profit from the proposed treatment, as is typically the case in medicine today. What I have seen is technology as a distraction from more effective ways to treat back pain that are slower, less profitable, and less glamorous.

Technology's impact on diagnosis and treatment goes even deeper. It actually alters the way that both doctors and patients think. This is no different than the arguments made about relying on GPS to get around our hometowns or the compulsion to check social media all day long. Technology has increased our appetite for distractions and medicine is not immune. The Internet, an ideal tool for learning, is instead merely used to acquire information. Gathering information is different than processing it. The doctor seems to speak to "a stranger in the room"—the computerized medical record system that exists in "the cloud"—necessitating a different language, motive, and mode of communication, which devalues the critical relationship between doctor and patient.

We are surrounded by the argument that medicine in America has to change. Our system is too expensive and not effective. And, in addition, it is actually causing harm. Doctors and patients are unhappy. Medicine is being invaded by technology. Medicine is becoming more of a business.

Back Pain Is My Guinea Pig

How we treat back pain serves as a prime example and metaphor for the current state of the American healthcare system. It is expensive, ineffective, and dangerous. As you will read in Part I: The Problem, it is my opinion that mostly proposed tests, diagnoses, and treatments are superfluous. The patient is often left unable to understand and work the system, which is not patient-centric or personalized but reliant on economics, metrics, and behavioral psychology. Most times back pain sufferers are led by their very providers through an arbitrary treatment driven by doing interventions—code for surgery, *unnecessary* surgery.

Although this seems like a harsh criticism, finding a different and better method of treating back pain may serve as a model for changes in the overall healthcare system. Strangely enough, I propose that a different model will circle back to the question of character, which will end up playing the most significant role in treatment of the spine.

Character in medicine looks no different than character that you seek out in a life partner, a friend, a teacher, or a babysitter. Providers must resurrect latent emotions and traits, natural and present but suppressed by the state of our current medical system, such as empathy and humility, and allow them to flourish and be communicated through the use of deliberate narratives. This means talking, listening, and engaging with one another's verbal and nonverbal cues. It has become a widespread talking point that families today are alone together on their gadgets in their own living rooms and dinner tables, and the same is happening in doctors' offices around the country.

At the same time, back pain sufferers will be required to participate in the changes. They will be asked to open their minds, become more autonomous in their decision-making, accept new ideas, admit to their expectations (fair or unfair), and acknowledge their existing biases about easy fixes such as medications or the overreliance in the belief that science has all the answers. All of this, too, will develop through the use of narratives: the patient's, the doctor's, and the doctor-patient narrative.

The end goal for the doctor will be to set his patients off on a journey of autonomy, whereby the patient becomes a partner in her healthcare, has choices and informed consent, feels her human rights are valued and that she is not merely representative of a dollar sign. In today's current treatment of back pain, patients arrive looking for something to be wrong with them and are dependent on the doctor's next steps. This is not indicative of a two-way narrative, but a one-way street that can lead only to more interventions. Despite the almost ubiquitous and urgent sense of a need for change, there is no real consensus as to what the change should be and how to go about making it. Additionally, the debate is politically charged and too early in its course to judge.

Medicine often appears polarized. Our healthcare is both the best in the world and quite poor, depending on how one chooses to judge it. Medical school admittance is as competitive as ever while doctors are at an all-time low in terms of job satisfaction.

Welcome to My Movement

The change that I have in mind is implemented one doctor at a time and one patient at a time. It does not rely on politics, lobbying, or top-down economics. As a plea to his doctor, essayist Anatole Broyard wrote in *New York Times* magazine, going on three decades ago,

> I wouldn't demand a lot of my doctor's time. I just wish he would brood on my situation for perhaps five minutes, that he would give me his whole mind just once, be bonded with me for a brief space, survey my soul as well as my flesh to get at my illness, for each man is ill in his own way . . . Just as he orders blood tests and bone scans of my body, I'd like my doctor to scan me, to grope for my spirit as well as my prostate. Without some such recognition, I am nothing but my illness.

What Broyard was saying in a nutshell is that he recognized his care was not optimal unless both the doctor and he developed and engaged in the active use of personal and cooperative narratives. Just as Broyard begged to have *himself* scanned, I call our solution to the problems of healthcare keeping the *me* in medicine—the deliberate development of ideas, stories and personal connections that facilitate medical care, encourage doctor-and-patient-centric strategies and outcomes, and develop and build character. On the surface, this solution looks like it has nothing to do with disease at all.

During my interview with The Monocle, I was asked whether an adult could alter his character. The question presupposes a yes or no answer. This book is about using narratives to find our personal shade of gray in a world demanding black or white. It is about pressing doctors and patients on their ability, need, and even desire to undergo a transformation in their character by embracing and sharing empathy, compassion, rhetoric, writing resources, and communication styles currently dropped from the system. Do you want to change in order to change the system? Answering "no" ensures that all we will be left with is a continuation of a go-nowhere, politically charged, finger-pointing, distracting, disagreement on how to run the healthcare system.

It sounds old-fashioned, ideological even, but this book aims to argue how these truths are the traits of a successful movement. Slow-and-steady, word-of-mouth, building-block types of implementation will help the ground to swell. My movement involves the use of narratives by both doctor and patient, to be used first individually and then in conjunction.

For doctors, it is the development of character through introspection and the application of that character into practice patterns. It is developed, not only from introspection, but from teaching, mentoring, or writing. It is a way of transcending the basic science of medicine and creating stories, analogies, anecdotes, or mental models, which will help the patient to understand more, to acquire health or to affect change. It is the development of ways to help patients contextualize their situations, and, in doing so, actually alter their health.

For the patient, it is a similar development of character that will allow for new mental models and habits that will similarly promote health.

The real power of narratives occurs when the doctor and patient are together and using technology cooperatively. The resonance between individually improved narratives allows for a new medicine. Combined narratives will not only create a dynamic form of expertise, it will change our traditional referral patterns and our methods of measuring value in medicine.

Narrative Medicine Is Not Novel

The power of the narrative has been recognized for centuries. Interest in the narrative has had a recent resurgence. Yale University's Department of Medicine holds a workshop to help doctors improve their skills as writers. In writing, doctors become better observers and thus better doctors. Columbia University has a master's program in Narrative Medicine. While it is obvious that the ability to act as a curator or creator of new and important information provides the patient with an invaluable service, the benefits for the doctor as a thought organizer, as a source of creativity, and as a way to reinforce one's own morality are less obvious. As Kierkegaard suggested, being ethical is to be the editor of one's life. Meditation is espoused at Stanford University as a method for not only improving healthcare providers' compassion, but also as a safeguard against provider burnout.

Why Bother?

I find myself working as a surgeon during the day, while at night and on weekends, I assume the role of protector of patients with back pain *from* surgeons.

How did I get here? Is it part of a masochistic desire to

cannibalize my career? I think that my Jekyll and Hyde nature has emerged from my similarly conflicted view of medicine, one filled with both awe and a sense that medicine is broken. This book offers my opinion on how to mend it and even improve it.

This treatment is more philosophical in nature and may seem strange coming from a surgeon. We, as neurosurgeons, after all, represent the epitome of specialization and technical prowess. But I believe, beyond technology and research and all of the great unknown scientific advances, it is the power of the narrative that needs to be taught and unleashed.

How to Use This Book

The book has been divided into four parts; the first begins the search to identify the hidden problems, what we don't know about how we got here in the first place. There are several smokescreens that have come along, such as medicalization and technology, which have on the surface seemed like progress but have, more times than not, detracted from good healthcare. In Part I, you will not only learn of the outside tangible forces like our overdependence on diagnosis and disease, the need for doctors to be right and feel important, insurance matters, the business of medicine, and the economics that contribute to the plight of the patient, but also of the more psychological and philosophical phenomena that infiltrate the ways doctors and patients relate to themselves and one another, alter the decision making process and cause bias and hubris, getting in the way of honesty, collaboration, accountability, and transparency.

After exploring the curious reasons providers and patients spiral deeper into a black hole, Part II begins to build the blocks of the promise ahead, particularly the traits, habits and end results of a system based on more human elements of character building, such as introspection, empathy, humility, embracing wrongness, understanding data and its skewing, better decision- making, self-policing, and shared decision- making and community. We will see how these building blocks transform how surgery is decided upon and performed, how well doctors and patients communicate their concerns, and how paternalism gives way to cooperative medicine.

Part III is heart of the book and focuses on the philosophy of narrative medicine, how to incorporate it into our personal lives, and how to use it to transform our doctor-patient relationships.

Finally, Part IV is the prescription to incite the narrative medicine movement. In the end, we will see that our problems have begun with us but that they can end with us, the doctor and the patient, by putting the *me* back in medicine.

My Wish

Returning to the ancient Indian parable speaks of a man with bare feet who wants to walk across a field of thorns and has two options: he can pave a path in the field or he can make himself sandals, In the preface, I suggested that this book is about changing ourselves—and it is. But something special occurs when we change ourselves, we change what is around us. If we each make a pair of sandals and walk together, we will also have paved a path in the field. If we change ourselves, we change the field of medicine.

PART I

THE PROBLEM

Inside You'll Find:

The Downside of Diagnosis and the Need for Disease

The Provider on the Pedestal

The Problems of Fee-for-Service Reimbursement and Insurance Providers

The Problem of Over Treatment

The Touchy Topic of Technology

I am sitting across the desk talking to a patient to whom I have just recommended surgery. She is distraught. But what is causing her such an emotional upheaval is not so much the fear of surgery itself. She is overwhelmed by the need to make a decision without the apparent information that she would suppose is necessary.

"How do I know whether you are the best one to perform this surgery?" she asks while I discuss possible surgery.

She's right. She has no good way to evaluate me. She can ask around, but that type of random sampling offers little real information. And yet, is of enormous comfort to many patients. Defying any logic, patients will routinely become enamored of a doctor after hearing only a couple of positive comments.

I often laugh to myself when I hear "how great I am" from a patient whom I have just barely met. Don't get me wrong, it feels great to hear it, but deep down I recognize that it has little meaning. I am tempted to ask, "How could you possibly know that?" Of course, I don't challenge my patients when they offer such praise because I know that their results will be better if they go into surgery with a positive feeling. That and it feels too good to correct. I would guess that the majority of surgeons believe themselves to be better than average—another defiance of logic.

Here's a simple question—and one without an easy answer: What makes a surgeon, or any doctor, good?

I occasionally feel that I'm inflicted with the "imposter syndrome," which tacitly affects many successful professionals. This syndrome leaves me with the feeling that I don't deserve to be a surgeon and that I will imminently be discovered by the "secret quality police."

When these feelings arise, I remind myself that I have arrived where I am as the result of sustained hard work and dedication. There is no shortcut to being a surgeon. Even those with extraordinary natural ability require years to achieve quality.

Surgeons occasionally engage in debates over what makes a surgeon good and why. While some suggest that being good is a function of hand dexterity or the understanding of three-dimensional anatomy, I believe that the answer lies in understanding the difference between an easy case and a case made to look easy. The surgeon is good if a case can be made to look easy. It's as simple as that.

If my patient were allowed into the operating room for a preview, her assessment of me would be more accurate. This is why the opinions of operating room nurses are so commonly solicited. They are thought to possess a sacrosanct insight.

Unfortunately, or really, fortunately, HIPPA precludes our patients grabbing a front row preview in the operating room.

Technical ability, though important, is not the overriding factor, particularly when most surgeons fall into an acceptable range. It is our humanity, and not our hands, that primarily define us as surgeons. Henry Ford once quipped, "Why is it every time I ask for a pair of hands, they come with a brain attached?" He looked at our humanity as being a detriment when standing as a cog in an assembly line. When it comes to surgery, I would ask the opposite, "Why every time a patient talks to a surgeon, the surgeon comes with a pair of hands attached?"

A surgeon with great results has been shown to lose this edge when operating in a different hospital. There is no difference in his technique in the alternative setting, but there is a different team. The power of a surgeon is partly in his capacity to assemble a team. Surgeons help their patients to decide. The prowess of a surgeon lies in his narratives as well as with his accumulated fund of knowledge or technical prowess.

This is what the patient across from me needs to understand.

In his book, *The Road to Character*, David Brooks contrasts resume virtues and eulogy virtues. The former contributes to ones "success" while the latter is emphasized at one's funeral. He suggests that our country has gone through a slow transformation to where we prioritize resume virtues. Brooks extols the concept of self-respect. He defines this as different than self-confidence or self-esteem. It is earned not by being better than others, but by being better than each of us used to be.

Part of why I have chosen to write this book gets back to the question that my patient is tacitly asking herself while I talk about possible surgery. "How do I know whether he is the best one to perform my surgery?" You see, in this book, I explore a related question: *How do I know that I am the best one to do her surgery?*

Put another way, how good a doctor have I become? Have I become better than I once was?

One of my original motivating factors for becoming a doctor

was to avoid becoming a salesman. Ironically, after the long process of becoming a doctor, I realize that I am a salesman of sorts. The product that I sell, of course, is myself. So, I wonder, how good is my product?

In the coming pages I will admit to and expose the magic and mayhem of the way in which we practice medicine and receive treatment, arguing the need for a slow and steady, grassroots approach to becoming better doctors and better patients--embracing our humanness and our innate need to connect on deeper levels than we are. In other words, we must find a way to keep the *me* in medicine. But first, let's look at the problem.

The Problem

I'm not about to reiterate the negativity that pervades the experiences of both doctors and patients today. I have written this book and you are reading it because we are in agreement that medicine is too expensive, that fee-for-service (doctors getting paid for doing something—or anything—even unnecessary things) is flawed, and that illness and morbidity caused by treatment or a physician is an issue. That's the stuff we already know. What the following addresses are the ideas, beliefs, behaviors, and habits that we have voluntarily opted for, but which are the real culprits to the disaster that is our healthcare system.

For instance, if I write that diagnosis can do more harm than good, that technology undermines the effectiveness of proper care *and* empowers it, that doctors routinely take credit for the placebo effect, and that it is surgeons' humanity—not their hands—that patients should be seeking, you might call me a lunatic. And I understand why. After all, it is difficult to accept that we have all been indoctrinated into a system that benefits the provider over the patient. It is human nature to want to *not* peek behind the curtain, because even though we want to "see," we might not feel equipped to adequately deal with what we find. And, additionally, we may discover that doctors may not want to alter a status quo that benefits them financially.

In an attempt to stop the insanity, Part One is a peek behind the curtain that masks the problems I have uncovered throughout my thirty years of being a surgeon which are only getting worse as time passes. The only way to be equipped to finally make positive changes to our healthcare system is for both doctors and patients to acknowledge the problems and be accountable to them, which in turn becomes part of the solution. That means, *we* are the solution.

Albert Einstein said, "If I had an hour to solve a problem, I'd spend fifty-five minutes thinking about the problem and five minutes thinking about solutions." This is precisely why we must begin with the problems and where we will spend much time uncovering them—the science, psychology, and business motivations behind them—which will make clear the things we need to do, practice, and implement in order to *become* the solution.

CHAPTER 1

The Downside of Diagnosis and the Need for Disease

John's back pain began to take over his life. It was his first thought every morning when he struggled out of bed. It was what he discussed with his friends. It was the source of fighting with his wife. John had a sense that people began avoiding him. He knew they didn't want to hear about how crummy he felt. He didn't want to talk about it either, but he was no longer able to work because of the pain and so he felt the need to justify himself.

His wife had lost patience with John. She was an empathetic soul, but couldn't understand why he couldn't simply deal with the pain and get back to work. She knew other people who worked with chronic pain. He had become a different person than the one she had married. Once the rock in her life, John now appeared feeble and needy.

John had seen several different specialists. Each had promised him that they could make him better and yet nothing had worked. Ultimately, he had been sent to a pain management doctor. While the decision to treat the pain may seem prudent, pain management often functions as a dumping ground for patients who are deemed not helpable. This doctor told John that the other doctors, by not sufficiently treating his pain early in its course, had enabled the growth of a pain pattern. He prescribed narcotic pain medications.

At first, the drugs helped, but now John was not so sure. His wife thought that the medications had further "changed" John and this added to their deteriorating relationship.

Finally, still searching for both a diagnosis and a solution, John sought out a rheumatologist who told him he had fibromyalgia, an autoimmune disease. While there is no blood test or scan to make this diagnosis, John's sensitivity to palpation of his muscles was the hallmark of the disease. The rheumatologist confidently told John that he was certain of the diagnosis.

He suggested an antidepressant. Although John didn't want to add another medication, he obliged, secretly thrilled with the diagnosis because, finally, he had an explanation for his pain. His wife and friends had doubted him—he had doubted himself—and now he was vindicated. This is why he couldn't work. This is why he wasn't himself. Sure, this was his plight in life, but at least there was a reason he felt the way he did.

But, is the diagnosis of fibromyalgia a *good* thing in this setting?

Fibromyalgia is a controversial disease for several reasons. First, no conclusive reason has ever been worked out to explain it. Second, the disease is associated with many bad situations: inability to work, difficult family life, chronic pain, medication addiction, etc. Third, diagnosis is often subjective and, even the objective criteria of diffuse hypersensitivity—the muscle palpitation John described—used to make the diagnosis is fairly subjective.

Are there advantages to a diagnosis of fibromyalgia? The disease provides the organizational structure to fund research or to do data analysis. The diagnosis provides Internet portals for patients with similar symptoms to exchange successes with medications, therapies, or other interventions. The diagnosis provides the patient with a sense of vindication. "There is a *reason* for me to have been complaining all of these years," John says. Finally, a diagnosis gives the doctor a way of finishing the office visit. Once the patient has been told that the diagnosis is fibromyalgia and that there is no proof and no ideal treatment, there can be closure to the patient's search for answers and the actual office visit.

At the same time, there are disadvantages. Once there is a diagnosis, costly treatments with little efficacy will follow. Some of these treatments will carry with them dangerous side effects, introducing more side effects and more cost. The patient may succumb to the chameleon effect—when patients begin to manifest symptoms of a disease simply because they now think they have the disease. This definitely happened to John, who began to walk slower, bend more carefully, and interpret every ache he felt as part of his diagnosis. He literally became a fibromyalgia sufferer simply because of the diagnosis he was given. Finally, a diagnosis can undermine the normal coping mechanisms that patients form for many of life's common symptoms, like muscle sensitivity and back pain.

If fibromyalgia is not a disease, these disadvantages represent what is known as the medicalization of some symptoms. Medicalization is a process by which conditions and problems that are characteristically a typical part of life come to be defined and treated as medical conditions, allowing them to become subjects of research study, diagnosis, prevention, or treatment. By definition, it is not a good thing. The explaining away of symptoms that are in some cases inevitable (e.g., degeneration) has been associated with the pejorative "disease mongering" that threatens the Me in Medicine and stands to sabotage the facilitation of doctor-patient narratives that are honest and transparent. In this case, the possible medicalization of John's diagnosis has the risk of undermining his coping mechanisms and redirecting the focus from coping to treating.

The world of back pain is a great example of a high demand for, and a need to offer, a diagnosis. While people who experience back pain are subjected to a variety of treatments such as chiropractic, anti-inflammatory medicines, different hands-on therapies, etc., none of the treatments have been shown to be effective when subjected to the scrutiny of evidence-based medicine, which emphasizes well-designed and well-conducted research. Does this mean that we don't have any good treatments for back pain, or rather, that the diagnosis "back pain" is many different things and thus counterproductive when used as an umbrella term? The jury is still out on this question, but the diagnosis of back pain, its presumed cause in each instance, and the justification to treat reigns supreme, despite the lack of demonstrated efficacy.

Now That I Know I Have Dis-ease, I Feel So Much Better

I would like to consider the conceptual use of diagnosis as a double-edged sword. Diagnosis provides patients a target to Google. It allows doctors and insurance companies to communicate what is being treated. Adding another statistic to a diagnosis can be used to raise money for research.

At the same time, disease can pigeonhole us into inappropriate treatments and burden us with counter-productive beliefs about our health and our limitations—the chameleon effect. Patients' descriptions are often quite broad and may intermingle and thus confuse one diagnosis with another that has shared symptoms. For example, low back pain is a symptom of both a kidney infection and a herniated disc.

Diagnosis is often made in the radiology suite or laboratory rather than at a bedside or in the office. Patients come into an office or hospital and a host of tests are ordered. These studies are admittedly spectacular. But here is what happens: they further distance the doctor from the diagnosis, which takes the personal relationship, the use of narratives, the practicing of cooperative medicine, and the chance to empower the patient away. As diagnosis becomes easier and more automated and more removed from the doctor, we cannot let the concept of diagnosis itself become empowered because that eliminates the Me in Medicine.

Our Need to Find a Reason

We are wired to have a why. When someone commits a heinous crime, we want to uncover a motive. When a spouse ends a marriage, the other needs to know the reason. When someone catches a cold, they wonder where they got it from or from whom they caught it. Everything is cause and effect, right? Black and white?

In medicine, there is a long history of assuming causation after finding a correlation. We, as doctors, have been taught to try and find a diagnosis or explanation in every setting. This is the reason why people are frustrated by new studies that say certain things are bad for health, only to hear a study a year later that reverses that information. This shows that we know that correlations are not the same as causations, but we continue to confuse the two. For instance, initially a correlation between colds and cold weather may be noticed because having a cold seems to occur more commonly in the winter. However, with the knowledge that a cold is caused by a virus, we can understand that in cold weather we tend to be crammed together indoors allowing for the transmission of the virus. Therefore, causation and correlation are not one in the same thing.

As patients, our desperation to have a "reason," is similar to the desperation of doctors to give one, and so we continue to spin our web to distract us from the truth: more times than we think, there is no cause, or, at least, none known. There isn't always black and white. We must learn to be comfortable with shades of gray. This gray area is important because, while it is true that establishing a cause can be a powerful conduit to better treatments which is part of the fabric of progress in medicine, confusing correlation with causation does just the opposite: creates confusion and overtreatment.

Nortin Hadler, M.D., Professor at University of North Carolina School of Medicine, refers to the pain that John was feeling as a predicament, which is neither cause or effect nor black or white. A predicament implies that there is a choice to be made. In the case of John's pain, his choice is to either tolerate the pain or to allow the medical system to mitigate the pain. In fact, in one of his papers "Low back pain: an intermittent and remittent predicament of life," Hadler writes, "For any of us to live a single year without a backache is abnormal. That is true throughout adult life. And that has, no doubt, always been true. What is mutable is whether, and how, and how well we cope with another such challenge to our sense of invincibility."

We have such predicaments all of the time. Maybe it is knee pain, neck pain, fatigue, etc., but the medical system has thrived financially by being the traditional option for patients with such predicaments, i.e., the medicalization of symptoms. In the case of John, and in the case of many of my patients, I have found this to not only be unnecessary, but harmful. Low back pain as a diagnosis is not helpful in that it both supposes a need to treat when it is a merely a common part of life, like a cold or headache, and it is also not specific enough to allow for a proven treatment. Subdividing back pain into subcategories, such as herniated disc or facet joint arthritis, won't solve the first problem (inappropriately suggesting that treatment is necessary) but may allow for more tailored and predictable treatments in the event that treatment is initiated.

In Part IV, The Prescription, you will discover the different narratives that help to embrace the reality of predicaments and, as Hadler advises, "cope with such challenge to our sense of invincibility."

John fell victim to the dependency of finding a why. While John's diagnosis of fibromyalgia did not lead to an adequate treatment, it served to *rationalize* his inability to work. It *justified* his persistent use of narcotic pain medication as well as antidepressant medication, both of which were having negative effects on his already declining relationships and on his personality. His diagnosis deprived him of his normal coping mechanisms.

Did the rheumatologist know this? Yes.

Then why did the rheumatologist make the diagnosis?

Because this is what doctors do.

CHAPTER 2

The Provider on the Pedestal

"**W**ould you tell your mother to have this operation?" This is a question I hear often and it is problematic for several reasons. First, there is the suggestion that the surgery I am recommending may be different than the suggestion I would give my mother, if the overall situation were comparable. That implies that my motive for suggesting the surgery may be self-serving and unnecessary. This inference is sad, not because it is an affront to my credibility, but because it is the tip of an iceberg that represents a justified general mistrust of medicine.

The second problem is that my patient's question presumes that there is a "correct" treatment and ignores the need for not the best treatment for a particular problem, but the best treatment *for a particular patient* with a particular problem. In other words, my mother and my patient may have the same problem, but there is no consideration that they may require different treatments because they are different people.

Finally, the question represents a cop out on the part of the patient. She looks to have me paternalistically make a decision for her with the benevolence that my mother would demand.

What appears to be a genuine question turns out to be an indictment of medicine. My patient views medicine as benefiting the providers more than the patients. And, she is right!

This is not a conspiracy, nor is the design intentional, but is the natural outcome of a system that has evolved over a couple of centuries. It is a system that has allowed itself to be derailed by the influence of business and technology. Just a couple of hundred years ago, medicine was practiced by not just doctors, but by a variety of healers without any training and in the individual households where the matriarch was often also the health provider. The consensus at that time was that medicine should not be the exclusive prowess of an elite profession, but available for anyone to learn and practice.

Slowly and steadily medicine became a profession, and then we put the provider on the pedestal. This process was undoubtedly bolstered by advances in technology and instrumental discoveries in medicine such as antibiotics and chemotherapy. Further bolstering medicine's role as a profession was the introduction of insurance companies, which became the method by which medicine was underwritten. These payments were available only to doctors, further bolstering their sovereignty. Most of medicine today is paid for by a fee-for-service method. In this model, doctors get paid based on how many patients they see or how many procedures they perform. Laboratories, X-ray facilities, and drug companies similarly get paid on how many tests, scans, or drugs they can muster. As a result, the very structure of the system has slowly evolved into a construct that demands more tests and interventions. It has also become an unsustainably expensive system.

It is not only the patients that are dissatisfied.

It doesn't take more than a couple of minutes of sitting in the doctor's lounge in a hospital to recognize the rampant dissatisfaction that underlies the practice of medicine. Doctors are being squeezed. Much of this is our own fault. We are a fiercely independent group that has survived years of pressure to gain a spot in medical school, years of sleep deprivation and scrutiny while training to be a doctor, and then, years of a system that often makes mistakes feel like crimes. Perhaps, as a result, we have felt like we are especially deserving and we have, thus, failed to adequately police ourselves.

We have substituted financial rewards for charitable rewards. We have failed to embrace and take advantage of communication technologies and systems that ensure safety. We find ourselves in the role of co-conspirators in the current epidemic of hospital acquired morbidity and mortality. The doctor, once revered, increasingly finds himself portrayed as money hungry, dishonest, and to blame for the dangers in medicine that are increasingly being exposed. We are active contributors to the waste.

The Origins of Waste

It has always fascinated me to trace back the path of a typical patient with back pain. The starting point is often arbitrary. Perhaps one's neighbor is a chiropractor or one's daughter is a physician's assistant and so a patient begins there. At other times, patients with a long-standing relationship and trust in their primary care physicians will open a dialogue about their pain with them.

A person's entry point into the medical system should be a minor issue because once the initial provider understands what is wrong, a patient should be appropriately referred to the correct provider.

Or not!

One of the issues with medicine today is that the treatment that patients ultimately receive is dependent on where they start and not on what is actually wrong. Sounds crazy, doesn't it? Most patients are aware of this on some level, but end up trusting what they are told. It is essential to understand that if you go to a provider, *that* provider will likely find something to treat and *that* provider will view his own treatment as the treatment of choice. These providers are not necessarily being exploitative. The chiropractor truly believes in the power of chiropractic and the surgeon in the power of surgery. The barber similarly believes that short hair looks better than long hair.

In addition to being arbitrary, the patient's entry into the medical system is subservient in its nature, meaning the majority of patients enter with the mindset of having their problem solved by the practitioner. Regarding back pain, patients must be honest with themselves about whether they are seeking medical help to have their problem fixed or to understand what is wrong, accepting that nothing needs fixing (the predicament discussed in chapter 1) and that the office visit is more an affirmation of modifications of their life health plan?

In Alexis's case, she saw her internist. She was one of fifty patients the internist had that day. Alexis was eager to share with her doctor the details of what she was experiencing. She wanted him to listen carefully, make a diagnosis, and then have him send her to the most appropriate and talented specialty provider. That was her plan.

But the internist was caught up in his own mess. He was stressed for time. He craved a quick solution to Alexis's problem, but also knew that there was no quick solution. He could take one of a couple of paths: He could refer Alexis to a specialist or he could manage Alexis himself and give her advice like go to physical therapy, lose weight, exercise, etc. If the internist referred her to a specialist, he would be acting in a cost-inefficient manner, because the cost of her care would be increased with more treatments likely ordered by the specialist. If the internist managed the case himself, though, Alexis would be denied the advantages of the specific expertise of a specialist.

The internist recommended an MRI of Alexis's lumbar spine and physical therapy. The MRI was done within a day, but Alexis had no access to the report. Diagnosis would have to wait until she saw the internist again. When she saw the internist, she was only read the conclusion from a radiologist's written report. Talk about isolation and glorification of the diagnosis. This process allowed the internist to charge for another visit (wasteful), and it separated the diagnosis from the clinical situation the patient was experiencing.

How meaningful was that report?

If you show a single MRI to three different radiologists, you may get three different reports. Even more remarkably, if you show one radiologist the same MRI at three different times, you may also get three different reports! This is not a criticism of radiologists, but a reminder that interpretation is human and thus subject to bias, subjectivity, and change. Or, in other words, the report is somewhat arbitrary. On top of this, there is no standardization in language, so what is a herniated disc to one radiologist may be a degenerative disc to another. Finally, abnormalities on MRIs are common—even when done on patients without pain.

Alexis's physical therapist seemed knowledgeable. She also had the results of the MRI report. "You have a herniated disc," she told Alexis. "I am going to start your therapy using the techniques of a physical therapist from New Zealand named Robin McKenzie." The physical therapist had extra training in this type of therapy and Alexis felt confident that it would make her feel better.

What the physical therapist didn't tell Alexis was that she had not read the MRI, but only the radiologist's report of the MRI. So, the internist and the physical therapist had read only the report of the MRI, and not the MRI itself!

Should Alexis still have felt so confident?

It turns out that, in this setting, the report is not as important as one would think. The current medical literature does not provide the therapist with a proven best treatment, as demanded by evidence-based medicine. Even if the MRI had provided the definitive cause of pain (the *why*), our current medical system does not know what the optimal treatment is for that condition.

What we do know is that the majority of patients with acute back pain will improve—with or without treatment. Patients come into the medical system believing that the treatments offered lead to the improvement that is ultimately experienced, but this is not necessarily the case. There is something called the "natural history" which is how the problem is likely to unfold without treatment, which is why patients should inquire about what would happen without treatment, which we will discuss again in chapter 17. Just as a provider will be biased toward a certain treatment, so will they be skewed in their own anecdotal evidence of improvements through such treatments. The perspective of the provider is determining the "science."

Alexis's therapist had opted to use McKenzie PT. It would have been preferable, however, to have had her look at the MRI first, as all disc herniations are not the same. In Alexis's case, the disc was not herniated, but rather, degenerative. Furthermore, it is impossible to know whether that degenerative disc was the cause of Alexis's pain. Most degenerative discs do not cause pain. Most are the result of a genetic predisposition rather than the result of an injury or excessive wear and tear.

If he had examined the MRI herself, Alexis's internist would have had the opportunity to explain that the disc abnormality found on the MRI was not important. Not important, because it likely had little to do with the pain, and even if it did, it was unlikely to improve from being "fixed." Instead, the internist told Alexis that her pain was coming from the disc.

Why did the internist so cavalierly hand out the diagnosis? The reasons are complicated. Doctors feel the pressure to supply an answer. If we don't supply it, the patient will think us unworthy or go to another physician. The patient expects an answer. Giving an answer lets the patient know that we are listening and we care. Offering an answer provides closure. A diagnosis produces a code that can allow reimbursement from the insurance company. Finally, the diagnosis forms the organizational structure that paves the way for subsequent treatments. Did the diagnosis add anything in this case? On the negative side, it added cost, misdirection, loss of coping, and pigeonholing of the patient's thought process, but, on the positive side, it increased doctor self-satisfaction.

Interestingly, the internist had supplied the therapist with the original prescription for physical therapy. In other words, the internist was telling the therapist what therapy to do. Not only had the internist not read the MRI, but he knew next to nothing about the practice of physical therapy. Therapists are given prescriptions by providers who know nothing about physical therapy; this is repeated daily in the world of physical therapy. Luckily therapists typically ignore the instructions and do what they think is best!

So, in a nutshell Alexis's experience went something like this:

Alexis developed back pain.

She was seen by an internist, who is not an expert in back pain and who was motivated to move her through the office visit as quickly as possible.

Alexis got an MRI, which was read by a radiologist who never saw her. The radiologist's reading was arbitrary but nonetheless used as a basis for the prescription from the internist, who wrote the prescription despite knowing nothing about therapy.

The therapist ignored the prescription, but also used the arbitrary MRI report to decide on a treatment, which was, in retrospect, wrong.

In addition to all of that, none of the providers, or for that matter, even an expert, could have "known" from where the pain was arising because the origin of back pain is typically indeterminable through an MRI of the spine.

Other than all of that, the system served Alexis well!

Neither the patient nor the various providers were satisfied. The process is time consuming, expensive, self-serving, and ineffective. Alexis did get better with the physical therapy, but this was in spite of the system and likely more attributable to the natural history of back pain and the innate capacity of the body to heal itself. The system took credit for Alexis's improvement and Alexis was pleased. She credits medicine with making her better. The provider is back on the pedestal, and it is up to the provider to figure out how to stay there.

How the Art of Misdirection Sustains the Illusion

One of the secrets of all good magicians is the art of misdirection. Sleight of hand is facilitated by having the attention of the audience briefly directed elsewhere. Of course, at a magic show, we are willing participants who find joy in being tricked.

In medicine, a similar misdirection often occurs. In this case the participant is a patient who would find little joy in such a distraction—if he or she were aware. This medical sleight of hand involves the manipulation of language rather than cards or coins. In this setting, the doctor is the magician and he, as well, may not be aware of the tricks being performed. Sometimes the trick is to introduce language that the patient doesn't understand. Other times, the question answered is different from what was asked. Whichever technique is chosen, the desired result serves the doctor—either by saving time, or, more likely, by avoiding saying three humiliating words, "I don't know."

My favorite analogy to this verbal trick can take place in your home. Your young child asks you, "What is sex?" You answer, "Sex is your gender. You are either male or female."

Definitely an answer—and an answer to the question asked—but not really the answer that your child seeks.

Guess what! Your child is often satisfied.

In the office, patients often ask me "Why does my back hurt?" I could say it's due to degenerative disc disease (after all, the MRI shows degenerative disc disease) but that would fall into the category of a true answer, albeit, a true and unrelated answer, similar to the answer about sex.

I could say that everyone's back hurts, but this avoids the "my" part of the question. I could suggest that the pain is muscular in origin. That's a great answer because it sounds authoritative and can't be proven or disproven. My favorite answer is "because you're overweight." That answer is not only unsubstantiated, but puts the patient on the defensive and therefore has the added benefit of ending the conversation quickly. After all, an overweight patient would never argue that he is not overweight.

What I should answer, of course, is that I don't know. The origin of back pain defies, more often than not, a definitive explanation. The good news is that it usually gets better. The patient should be told not to waste time on a question that can't be answered and simply return to his routine as tolerated.

"I don't know" is tough to say because the patient expects an answer from the doctor. Similarly, the doctor feels the pressure to provide an answer. The real answer is time-consuming. Here's where the magic of misdirection comes in. The verbal sleight of hand allows the doctor to give an answer, save time, and avoid those humiliating three words "I don't know." Misdirection is a problem because, while it saves time, it undermines the information that the patient seeks and can potentially benefit from.

Similar scenarios play out every day in the world of healthcare. While it is easy to blame doctors for being arrogant, part of the issue is that the doctors have traditionally owned the information and positioned themselves as the sole purveyors of that information. For this reason, they are not often challenged, and the distinction between what is proven and what the doctor simply believes becomes blurred.

In a well-known experiment, a group of participants were asked to watch a video where players, wearing white-and-black T-shirts, passed around a basketball. The participants were asked to count the number of passes made by the white T-shirt players. Halfway through the video, an actor in a gorilla suit walked across the screen. After the video, when asked if they saw anything out of the ordinary, more than half of the participants failed to mention the gorilla. Yes, we are very susceptible to, and unsuspecting of, misdirection.

My narrative is to embrace the answer "I don't know" because misdirection is a form of dishonesty.

Another form of misdirection is blaming the patient. It works, and I see my surgical colleagues pull it off. "Your surgery has an eighty percent chance of success," says the surgeon. Depending on your perspective, this may be good or bad. I am often shocked that some patients are overwhelmingly pleased while others are actually mortified by this same statistical prediction of success. It depends on what your expectations are prior to coming to see the surgeon.

Let's assume that the statistic of 80 percent is correct. Let's also assume that the surgeon performs several cases like this a week. Over a year, that results in a significant number of patients who are unhappy with their surgery.

How does the surgeon deal with these patients? No surgeon wants dissatisfied patients returning to the office stating that the surgery was not successful. The surgeon does not want his office hours to be cluttered with such discontents. This would leave less time to book new surgeries. It would also expose the new patients to those discontented patients in the waiting area—not good for business. The surgeon must develop a way to dismiss them and that's where the blame game begins.

Exposing the Secret Art of Dismissal

This marvel of dismissal involves a two-step process. The best in the business are able to not only dismiss the patient, but also, leave the patient blaming himself. First, the surgeon introduces the possibility of failure with the surgery. This is done prior to the surgery and clearly enough to be heard and referenced later, but timed just after the patient has made the emotional commitment to surgery; this way, the possibility of failure will not dissuade the patient from undergoing the proposed surgery.

The second step occurs after surgery. The patient is reminded that the possibility of failure had been stated explicitly before the surgery. In addition to that, there are several ways that the surgeon can blame the patient for the failure. "You produced too much scar tissue"; "You are overweight"; and the classic, "You didn't follow my directions." If the surgeon is really an artist, the patient in pain will apologize to the surgeon for undermining the surgery.

The less nuanced surgeons have less subtle techniques of dismissal. In this regard, self-delusion can be very helpful. One of my favorites is the surgeon who looks at the postoperative X-rays in front of the patient and says, "It looks good. I can't imagine why you have pain," as if it was only the execution of the surgery and not the rationale for the surgery that was relevant. Success requires both good indications and good execution; doing the wrong procedure leads to bad results.

And, on the other end of the spectrum, we have the bulldogs, where subtlety is not even considered. This is best accomplished by the surgeon stating (typically without eye contact and as he is exiting the room) that the job was done correctly and then allowing his office staff to tell the patient that the encounter is over. Often a physician's adjutant such as a physician's assistant or nurse practitioner is given this unenviable task.

The art of dismissal has grown out of our fee-for-service healthcare system. Surgeons that are willing to prioritize profit need to find ways to continue their practice without getting bogged down. A system where the doctor gets paid for value rather than procedure will obviate the need for dismissal. Such a system will quickly limit the number of unnecessary surgeries performed. In this system patients will still have to apologize to their surgeons but that apology will occur because the surgeon is not being paid for his hard and not meaningful work. It is easy to blame the doctor in these scenarios, but the problem is not the doctor. The vast number of doctors are well-intentioned. It is the system that ultimately corrupts the process. The system has been constructed to benefit the providers and not the patients.

CHAPTER 3

The Problems of Fee-for-Service and Insurance

Adam's pain returned and he came to see me as a "last resort." He had been living with back pain for years. Over that time, his pain had steadily worsened and his repertoire of activities had narrowed. Adam is not the type of person to passively accept such a fate, and so, he had tried many potential solutions. He had tried chiropractors, physical therapists, a host of medications, various injections, and even behavioral therapy.

Adam had a strong bias against surgery, but was at his wit's end. After I took a history and did an examination, we looked at his MRI together. Adam had degenerative disc disease at the bottom of his spine. More specifically, his L5-S1 labeled disc space had lost water content and height. The rest of his spine was relatively pristine.

I explained to him that although it was logical to assume that this rotten looking disc was the cause of his back pain, there was plenty of literature showing that surgical treatment in this setting was, by and large, disappointing.

Adam understood this, but his own sense of desperation forced him to pursue the conversation. He asked me if surgery *could* improve his pain.

My answer, "It could, but it is not predictable enough to warrant surgery in my opinion" was not satisfactory to him. He returned with, "What if I want to take that risk?"

This is a fairly common scenario that I face in the office. Further complicating the scenario is the added burden of convincing the insurance company to pay for the surgery.

Insurance companies are in the business of making money. Several years ago, after oncologists had some success in treating blood cancers with bone marrow transplants, there was understandable interest in extending the technique to other cancers such as metastatic breast cancer. This particular treatment is very dangerous to the patient and requires first the intentional destruction of the immune system and then replacement of a new immune system from a donor.

At the time, bone marrow transplant was being offered by oncologists to their metastatic breast cancer patients even though there was no good evidence to support its efficacy. The patients had been given a death sentence and were desperate and justifiably wanted to give it a try. The treatments were also extremely expensive and the insurance companies were also justifiably hesitant to underwrite something that wasn't "proven."

Not unexpectedly, lawsuits were filed and the insurance companies capitulated after suffering some large payouts and worrying that their image would be further tarnished. Ultimately, when studies were done, a lack of evidence permitted the insurance companies to deny payment.

Today, this tension is played out on a daily basis. What is at stake here is not life and death, but quality of life. The same question is posed, however: Should insurance companies underwrite a procedure that might help, but, statistically, has not been shown to help when viewed over a population of patients. Let's say that the predicted success rate is only 50 percent. Should Adam be given the chance to have the surgery if he is willing to take the risk? Since the operation is so expensive, the insurance company's refusal to pay is, in effect making the decision for the patient.

There are lots of ways to look at this question, but let me start by saying that if we are going to put the Me in Medicine, then the insurance company should not be part of the decision process. Of course, it's not so simple. Often, the insurance company conveniently blends the concepts of "no evidence to support" and "evidence of no support." I am often forced to speak with an insurance doctor on the phone to gain permission. I am told that there is no evidence to support a particular surgery. There is little evidence-based support for many things we do in life. Parachutes have never been proven as necessary accessory gear when jumping out of planes, but I would recommend wearing one if you like jumping out of planes. It is far too time-consuming and expensive to produce evidence-based support for everything. More significantly, if the proposed procedure for Adam had a relatively low chance of success and Adam was willing to take that chance, is it fair for the insurance company to deny him the chance? This is an example where the surgeon is pushing for a procedure (fee-for-service incentive) and the insurance is pushing against the procedure (claiming lack of evidence, but in reality, trying to save money).

What about Adam?

As a surgeon I have worked very hard to transcend the bias to do surgery. This is part of my narrative. As John and I sat and contemplated surgery, we attempted to make a decision together. This decision was an integration of my knowledge base and experience and his personal preferences and consideration of his life flow. This is a potent collaboration. In this case, the insurance company's refusal to pay negated our combined power.

The Business of Medicine

The cost of catastrophic healthcare will never be affordable to the unlucky individual who needs extensive care. There will, therefore, always be a need for some kind of insurance. Current reimbursement methods have converted medicine into a kind of assembly line where the meaning has been sapped from the individual encounters between doctor and patient. Although I would rather focus on how medicine is practiced than how it is paid for, the two are inseparable.

Perhaps even more regrettable than the way a fee-for-service payment increases costs is the way it pits the doctors who are motivated to do more tests and procedures against the insurers who are motivated to do fewer tests and procedures. The result of this conflict is that both doctors and insurers lose sight of doing what is best for the patient.

Blue Cross/Blue Shield in North Carolina recently decided it would not pay for spinal fusions for degenerative disc disease. This operation has long been a focus for me because it seems to be the most significant source of the bad reputation that spine surgery has come to bear. The operation has the dubious distinction of being largely ineffective and commonly performed—a bad combination indeed!

But, despite this, what are we to make of a unilateral decision of an insurance company not to pay for a particular operation? Following this decision, the number of fusion surgeries has diminished in North Carolina. Since this is generally not a good operation we must interpret the decision of Blue Cross/Blue Shield as good, shouldn't we?

The real issue is that the decision by the insurance company is largely motivated by cost. It is a reminder that the goals of any insurance company are not only misaligned with the providers, but also with those of the patient.

Similarly, what are we to make of the surgeons who perform these surgeries? These surgeons are motivated by the desire to make their patients feel better, but are also motivated by the fees that they receive in exchange. Again, the goals are not aligned with those of the patient, who simply wants to feel better. You can see how the business of medicine can interfere with the practice of medicine.

Perhaps it is with Big Pharma that the business of medicine appears most distressing. The pharmaceutical industry is responsible for some of the most amazing advances in medicine. If it is not allowed to profit, the means for such progress will be stifled. Americans pay double per capita the average cost for their prescription drugs. This is rationalized by the pharmaceutical industry as necessary for the research and development needed to bring new drugs to market. However, these same companies often spend more on marketing than they do on research and development.

You know that medicine has become too much of a business when convincing one to use a medication is prioritized relative to making the medication effective. There have been instances where the industry held back on disclosing side effects of the medications because such information would interfere with a successful marketing campaign. Finally, there is the relationship of any business with politics. Millions are spent in political contributions and political lobbying making it impossible for politicians to interfere with the actions of Big Pharma.

In the interest of business, doctors do not want to be scrutinized. In the book *Unaccountable: What Hospitals Won't Tell You and How Transparency Can Revolutionize Health Care*, Martin Makary tells the story of a Dr. Hodad. The fictitious last name is an acronym for "hands of death and destruction." This doctor is dangerously bad, and yet, no one is willing to call him out on it. What makes the story so scary is that when the narrator finally meets this infamous legend, he is blown away—not by his rude and crude manner, which is how he had envisioned him—but by an affect that is treacherously charming. One feels dreadfully sorry for his patients.

Equally disconcerting to me is the thought that doctors relate to the story because we all have experienced other doctors who we not only wouldn't send our families to but who we judge as incompetent. And yet, we doctors don't take action. Such action would be time-consuming and socially damaging—a form of political suicide. Let's face it, there is a bit of a boy's club in medicine. Besides, we rationalize our passivity with the philosophical position of "Who am *I* to judge competency"?

Medical boards and other regulating bodies arose from the deliberate desire of doctors to be distinguished from lay practitioners. This process has provided sovereignty to doctors and a degree of authority. It is no accident that the term used to describe the written suggestion of the doctor in a hospital is an "order."

With authority comes responsibility and our boards should be more aggressively involved in self-policing, but they are comprised of doctors and, thus, notoriously lenient. Restraint of trade is considered a harsh response to doctor inadequacy and usually applied only to outright corruption.

We occasionally have the desire to re-direct our patients when we don't approve of a peer's management or ability. This is often done surreptitiously as it is generally felt to be socially inappropriate. I am guilty of telling my patients "You may want to seek another opinion" rather than, "Your doctor sucks," and we often seek to further protect ourselves with "Remember, that suggestion didn't come from me."

The business of medicine leaves doctors resistant to transparency, even though we know that such transparency will make us better. When New York State published the mortality statistics for cardiac surgeries, what followed was a clear and sustained improvement in the quality of the hospital cardiac programs. Those which were below average either changed or disappeared.

When a patient with a back problem gets an MRI or lab test, he is often asked to return to the office to go over the report. This is an example of using information to extract a fee. This is a reasonable component of any business, particularly if the information is accompanied by teaching or advice. But what happens when the information can be directly accessed by the patient and the visit is no longer necessary for the purposes of getting the information? What happens when the patient decides that advice on the Internet or in an online back pain discussion forum is more valuable than that given by the doctor?

Today's doctor seems likely to order the diagnostic blood tests or imaging study so that the diagnosis can be made in a lab or the radiology department. In this setting, the doctor devolves from the diagnostician to the mere purveyor of the diagnosis. If the doctor himself limits to this role, he will soon be vulnerable to the process called disintermediation, the elimination of the "middle man" when the middle man is no longer essential.

Disintermediation is a phenomenon that has affected many of today's industries. A good example is with the realtor or car salesman. At one time, these professions enjoyed a body of knowledge that the customer didn't have access to. The business of real estate or car sales exploited this imbalance of information as a source of income. As the Internet evolved, so did the customer's ability to acquire information. The realtor and car salesman needed to establish some other role to provide the customer with value. Those who tried to hold onto the old system became obsolete.

Doctors are on the proverbial chopping block as well. Doctors will no longer be able to make a living as purveyors of information but will need to find another valuable function to offer. They often find it by treating things that don't necessarily need treatment.

CHAPTER 4

The Problem of Overtreatment

The assassination of President James Garfield is great example of the adage, no good deed goes unpunished. His gunshot wound should not have been a fatal one. His medical treatment was fatal, however. Because he was the President and deserved the "best" medical treatment, experts were brought in to use their hands to inspect the wound and search for the bullet. It was this excessive probing that likely introduced the bacteria that led to the sepsis that killed the President, rather than the actual gunshot.

We often refer to this as the VIP syndrome. When an "important" patient comes into a hospital, the "important" doctor is solicited to either do something he doesn't regularly do or simply to do something so that the important patient has been treated by the important doctor. The VIP syndrome often leads to worse medical care.

Medical treatment has become the leading cause of preventable death and disability in the United States. The medical industry is a parasite in the setting of overtreatment. At first glance, this is a frightening thought. But let's look at the automobile industry, which is also associated with a mind-numbing number of deaths. The convenience and advantages provided by cars force us to interpret the danger of driving as a necessary evil. No one is demanding the elimination of cars. Such is also the case in medicine. Progress will always come at a cost. There will always be morbidity and mortality associated with medical care. This is not to say that we shouldn't be obsessed with diminishing mistakes.

Eliminating mistakes in medicine starts with transparency. This transparency will need to be part of a larger cultural shift, which, like the aviation industry, uses mistakes as sources of growth and improvement rather than as punishable acts.

But before we get there, we must ask an even more basic question: what if the medical care provided is unnecessary? In this setting, unlike with the automobile industry, the complications should not be interpreted as a necessary evil.

The unnecessary care that has typically been discussed is that which comes at the end of life. Obviously, it is not always clear to the patient, the patient's family, or the doctor that the end of life is imminent. Such things become much clearer in retrospect. There is no doubt that patient and doctor narratives can alter this phenomenon. In *Being Mortal: Medicine and What Matters in the End*, Atul Gawande poignantly elucidates our cultural inadequacies in dealing with death. Patients who create narratives can articulate a priority for quality of life over simply living longer. Doctors will also serve as better contextualizers in this setting if they dedicate some deliberate time to forming their own end-of-life narratives.

More than unnecessary care at the end of life, there is a second example of unnecessary care that is often overlooked—medical care for the well. This is an area where we could, and should, ration care. This rationing should not consist of denials, but occur naturally with education. This will arise naturally from the narratives created by both patients and doctors.

The Institute of Medicine published a study in 2010 suggesting that 30 percent of Medicare spending was wasted—to the tune of 750 billion dollars. Half of this waste was accounted for by high prices, administrative costs, and fraud. Although I have no doubt that is true, I am interested in a different kind of waste. Not the waste of corruption and bureaucracy, which of course should be targeted, but a more treacherous waste—the medical care that arises from incomplete science and treatments that spring from the innocent sources of commonsense, habit, and tradition. I will use the term medicalization, again to encapsulate such unnecessary use of our resources.

Medicalization

In his book *The Citizen Patient: Reforming Health Care for the Sake of the Patient, Not the System,* Nortin M. Hadler, M.D., refers to the unnecessary use of resources as type II medical malpractice. Whereas traditional malpractice is described as doing what is necessary, poorly, type II medical malpractice is doing what is unnecessary, well.

Patients must understand they are victimized by today's medical system, which has been constructed by, and thus primarily benefits, the providers and not the patients. Education of both doctors and patients is the first step eliminating type II malpractice. It's not just a matter of making doctors and patients privy to the facts. It requires the creation of narratives that need to grow out of a deliberate introspection that questions the status quo.

Patients, who are the victims of type II malpractice, are ultimately responsible for digging themselves out from this tyranny, which is maintained not only from the expression of self-interest of the providers, but by the habits, predilections, and complacency of the patients themselves.

The Problem of Prevention

Everyone thinks that preventative medicine is ultimately more efficient than reactive medicine. One of the rationales for universal healthcare is to provide the opportunity for patients to be treated preventatively rather than coming into the emergency room floridly ill. An ounce of prevention is worth a pound of cure. One of the staples of preventative medicine is screening. It, too, has evolved into a process that can lead to unnecessary treatment.

Blood pressure is a great example. Science has demonstrated a definite advantage to reducing high blood pressure. What if your blood pressure is only a little bit high? The science is less convincing in this setting and thus rather than jumping into treatments with medications, trying dietary and exercise treatments should often be the patient's first move.

Blood pressure represents a reasonable screening candidate. It is cheap and reasonably reproducible and accurate. The trick with blood pressure is to treat that which is very high and be more circumspect with that which is borderline. Other forms of screening that are done in the spirit of preventative medicine are less clear. For example, screening for breast cancer, prostate cancer, and colon cancer can save lives, but at an expense. That expense is not simply cost. False positives can result in anxiety and stress, or worse, in unnecessary further testing and treatments, with their obligate complications and further cost.

Screening not only produces false positives, but true positives, of course. Cancer screening reveals cancers earlier than the eventual symptoms would reveal. Even when the screening successfully identifies a cancer, subsequent treatment is occasionally unnecessary for some of those cancers found. Additionally, the treatment at the earlier time provided by the screening doesn't always amount to better results. This is not to say that we should not screen, but that the process should be more circumspect than just looking at the number of positives acquired by the screening. In Part 4, I will describe how a doctor can form a narrative that will be essential when deciding whether to screen or not.

Bait-and-Switch Medicine

A police officer finds a man on his knees under a streetlight at night. The man is searching for his lost keys. The officer asks, "Are you sure you lost them here?" The man responds, "No, but I can see better here."

This is a great metaphor for action in medicine. We tend to pursue what is easiest rather than what is best for us. Similar to our tendency to use heuristics—mental shortcuts—as a substitute for difficult decisions, we prefer to obsess over surrogate markers over more holistic approaches to health.

When patients take a cholesterol drug, what they really want is to live longer and better. This association is difficult to prove and difficult to understand. Rather than adopt such a generalized purpose, the patient will focus on a particular number like cholesterol level. If the cholesterol has gone down, the patient is happy. This result is sufficiently satisfying as to preclude focusing on the more complicated issues. Much more difficult would be creating health habits that includes diet, exercise, and sleep. This requires a lot more work than taking a medication to keep cholesterol at a certain level. I'm not against lowering cholesterol, but when it serves as an isolated goal, it can, paradoxically, undermine health attainment.

Closely tied to over-focus on a lab value is the idea that action beats inaction. In this setting, actions serve as a surrogate for progress. As such, it can also paradoxically stifle progress. "Don't just do something, sit there." This clever reordering of words comes from John Bogle, the advocate of index funds as an investment vehicle. His premise is that an individual investor will do best by buying and holding passive collections of stocks that follow the market. Trying to frequently buy and sell generates income for the financial industry at the expense of the individual investor. Just as the financial industry can be conceptualized as a parasite in this analogy, so can the medical industry in the setting of overtreating.

Prioritizing action or what is easy may mean choosing to take a pill or have an operation. Similarly, easiest may also be reflexively doing what the doctor says. The patient must remember that the current system is constructed for the benefit of the providers. Some of what the doctor says may be based on things other than what is best for the patient. As discussed earlier, some doctors similarly feel the need to "do something" or perhaps the ambiguous literature suggests a possible benefit for a particular pill or perhaps that doctor has recently met with an attractive rep from the company that makes the pill. In this setting, the doctor may suggest the pill. This is not based on a strong conviction, but something somewhere between habit and guilt.

The company that produces the pill that has marginal benefit will also directly put pressure on the patient with advertisements or powerful testimonials. It is not uncommon to hear statistics such as "this pill will improve you by fifty percent." The circumspect patient will understand that much of the statistics provided are simply "noise." For example, when the incidence of a particular problem is low, a change of 50 percent or even 100 percent may be irrelevant. But it sounds impressive. In contrast, smoking increases the risk of lung cancer by 20to 30times or 2000-3000 percent. This is not noise and should not be ignored.

Doing something for the sake of doing something has a downside as well. It is interesting that when patients with terminal cancer are switched from chemotherapy to hospice care, they end up living longer. This underscores the idea that all treatments have a downside. If there is no proven upside, treatment can be worse than no treatment.

I believe that here is a place for action. After all, I am a surgeon. But action should not be initiated because it ought to be better than inaction. Embracing the world of gray without the need to act or decide between black and white will save money and result in better medicine.

CHAPTER 5

The Touchy Topic of Technology

When my friend drives to an unfamiliar location, she is totally comfortable. She mindlessly follows Google Maps and has no anxiety in finding her destination. Surely this is a technological advantage that saves time and frees her mind for a more meaningful brain utilization than navigation. The problem with my friend, however, is that she has no sense of where she is going. She can't visualize her trip from a 10,000-foot perspective. She can't even say that her destination direction is north or south. Perhaps most concerning is what is she capable of doing if the navigation system breaks.

Surgeons have the capacity to extract the data from an MRI or CT scan so that when removing a brain tumor. We can see a virtual image of the tumor as if looking through the side of the head. We no longer have to guess where to make the incision or how large to make the craniotomy (piece of skull bone removed). When I started in neurosurgery, part of the training was learning how to use visual and tactile landmarks on the scalp to help formulate the placement, shape, and size of the incision. New technology eliminates the need for this formulation. Incisions are smaller and effortlessly placed in an ideal location in today's operating room.

Surely, this is a good thing for the patient. But is losing the art of incision formulation good for the doctor? On the one hand, it frees up the doctor's mind to better focus on more important parts of the surgery. On the other hand, it allows for an acquired skill, a way of thinking, to fade away. In this way the surgeon's skill set is changed, in some ways, for the better, and, in other ways, in a diminished sense.

With every advance in technology, there is not only a gain, but something lost. For the most part, the gains outweigh the losses, but I am interested in looking at those arts that technology has taken from us. Spending some time mastering those arts, even if they are "unnecessary," has some value.

The airplane serves as a great example of technology viewed as a double-edged sword. As computers have increasingly become part of the control of a plane in flight, there have been obvious benefits in safety. While the computer has become an integral part of take-off, landing, and flight navigation, the pilot's role has been accordingly diminished to running the computer.

While this is a tribute to the computer's capabilities, the pilot's overreliance on the computer serves to erode his capabilities as a pilot. One has to wonder whether there will be skilled pilots left to guide planes in the event of a computer failure—or bird strikes! It is analogous to giving a back brace to a patient with back pain. At first, the patient feels better, but, in the long run, the brace weakens the core muscles and causes more back pain.

Computers undermine quality in other ways as well. With many different computers interconnected, a malfunction in one can sometimes cause a more systemic error that is hard to recognize or fix. This, coupled with an overreliance on computers, can result in more significant errors.

It is important to remember that computers can't think and that as good as they are at certain tasks, they are unable to display insight, humility, empathy, and many other human qualities that are often helpful in ambiguous situations or situations that are fickle or changing.

In addition to making us over reliant and diminishing our vigilance, computers can undermine our capabilities in an even more subtle way—by changing the way we actually think. Nicholas Carr, in his book *The Shallows: What the Internet Is Doing to Our Brains*, depicts the effects of the computer on the very fabric of our thinking. Just as the printing press profoundly changed the way we communicated, it also changed the way we would thereafter think. The world literacy rate dramatically rose with the availability of print. Perhaps this relationship between our media and how we think was best described by Marshall McLuhan with the pithy aphorism "the medium is the message." This idea from the 1960s encapsulates the far-reaching effects of the printing press and is still relevant today with regards to the Internet and other means of computer-driven communication.

As technology becomes more facile with image recognition, it is easy to imagine computers doing a better job of reading MRIs than humans. The computer will end up being more consistent and objective. In the not-too-distant future, if a patient develops a rash, a picture of the rash taken by the patient on a smartphone will be uploaded and diagnosed by a computer. It is easy to imagine a world in which the doctor is often bypassed.

Improved virtual reality will allow medical students to better learn anatomy. Surgeons will use the technology to practice their skills or to simulate surgery prior to the actual operation. This would mitigate one of the tensions that every surgeon faces—balancing the need to learn new things with the fear of making the patient the proverbial canary in the coal mine.

The future of medicine is exciting. Technology is going to continue to change medicine at a fast clip. I imagine that when I ask my near-future patient "Are you active?" he will not provide the meaningless, "Yes, I am very active." He will, rather, download his actual activity as derived from an accelerometer on his phone or watch. Technology, in the form of biosensors, will replace the subjective, descriptive parts of health with a quantitative representation that will be more accurate and usable. These data will be acquired automatically and effortlessly. We have the computer power now to not only manage this deluge of data, but to utilize it in a way that makes medicine more precise and better.

But when I walk onto a hospital floor I see the doctors and nurses gathered around the computer terminals and not next to the patients. Doctors' notes are reimbursed on the basis of how many "bullets" they contain. Such a system designed to encourage complexity and completeness paradoxically pulls the doctor away from the patient so that the note can be embellished. What was by design created to reward value ends up doing the exact opposite. Similarly, hospitals are paid, in part, on what is documented in the charts. As a consequence, the nurses' roles transition to document-ers and away from caretakers—just what the patients don't need or deserve.

Perhaps technology's tendency to separate the caretakers from the patients is most evident in the remarkable rising role of the radiologist as diagnostician. In the past, diagnosis was made at bedside. Just as Alexis's internist did, more and more, doctors sim-ply order lab tests and images and wait for the diagnosis to come back. These diagnoses are made in an Oz-like method, with the radiologist or laboratory hidden behind the curtain. Of course, this capability is a tribute to the improved sophistication of lab test-ing and the remarkable progress in imaging. The interpretation of MRIs and CT scans has become a super-specialized skill. The problem is that with the digitalization of images, the interpreta-tion of the tests take place in a part of the hospital isolated from the clinicians and patients. The super-specialized radiologist is not privy to the subtle aspects of the patient's clinical presentation. This introduces a systemic flaw—a disconnect—in diagnosis.

Similarly, electronic records add a new persona into the office or hospital visit, the computer. While the patient talks, the doctor types into and stares at a computer screen. The doctor and the patient end up competing for attention with the introduction of this third party. Even the product of the new guest, the medical record, has been devitalized. What was originally a contextual, creative piece of art is now a sterile, automated list and a bill generator, devoid of originality and spirit. The final note may be longer with more apparent information, but the ability to paste or use templates leads to a sterile note, devoid of character and unable to convey the subtleties and other "human" aspects of the encounter. Just as "cut and paste" has eroded our children's capacity to research and write a paper in school, it has eroded the value of the medical record. Each technological advance must be accompanied by a deliberate effort to maintain our humanity, the Me in Medicine.

In chapter 9, we will offer the prescription, the narrative, for enhancing the gifts technology gives us and safeguarding from the pitfalls of technology as just discussed.

We turn to the part of the book that deals with solutions. This is the promise portion, what medicine can and will be like. The solutions are simple, but not easy. Let's embrace the shades of gray and be ready to grow and change.

PART II

THE PROMISE

Inside You'll Find:

The Promise of Empathetic Paternalism

The Promise of Better Decision-Making

The Promise of Patient Autonomy

The Promise of Technology

The Promise of the Placebo

The Red Queen is a character in Lewis Carroll's *Through the Looking-Glass.* In the story the Queen is pushing Alice to run faster. When Alice realizes that she is running but remaining in the same spot, the Queen tells her that to in order to make progress she needs to run "twice as fast as that."

What if I told you that the messes we've made of medicine, the problems as I have presented them in the last section, could be mitigated—that the promise for living a life filled with prevention, health, and vitality are within reach.

This will require equanimity rather than the frantic approach of the Red Queen. You will be asked to accept predicaments of symptoms and consider treatments with less impulse and more thoughtful action. Medicine is in constant flux and requires action, but still, what if I told you that the promise of becoming better patients and becoming better doctors is nothing like running frantically (simple but aimlessly), but a rather calm and methodical approach.

My question "What if I told you," is no longer hypothetical; it actually never has been. As you turn the page to Part II: The Promise, I will show you what the future of medicine can look like. It is a future that values learning over accumulating facts, the acquisition of medical mental models to help us process our health concerns and to make decisions, and the adaptation of healthy habits. It is a process where patients become more autonomous and, strangely enough, where doctors become more paternalistic—not the old-fashioned and self-serving paternalism, that was part of the problem outlined in Part 1—by returning to an empathetic relationship paradigm between doctor and patient, known as empathetic paternalism.

CHAPTER 6

Empathetic Paternalism

Early in my career, I consulted on Miriam, who had a brain tumor. The tumor was adjacent to her left hemisphere and had produced a considerable amount of brain edema (excess water and swelling of the brain). The patient had developed what was described as confusion (more appropriately categorized as difficulty with language) and mild right-sided weakness.

After taking her history, examining her, and reviewing her MRI, I discussed with Miriam treatment options. I explained to her that the tumor warranted treatment. I discussed both radiation and surgery and recommended the latter, due to the size and accessibility of the tumor. I explained that I thought the tumor was benign and could be safely removed.

As I have committed to keep natural histories of conditions a part of my narratives, we discussed how her condition would progress without surgery, which I anticipated would be a progressive loss of language function and progressive weakness. This enabled me to present to her, with transparency, the depth of her condition and allow her to see the picture as broadly as possible.

Looking back, what all of this really meant was I that wanted her to see the condition the way *I* saw it.

With almost no hesitation, Miriam told me that at eighty-two, she was too old for surgery. She wanted to die with dignity and did not want to have any surgery at this stage of her life.

Because I strongly disagreed with her decision, I stated my case more emphatically. She stood her ground, and I realized that more discussion would be in vain. Later, I contacted her next of kin—two granddaughters living in Boston and Washington. Via conference call, I told them I believed their grandmother was making the wrong decision and that I felt strongly about the need for surgery.

Ultimately, the granddaughters gained power of attorney and authorized the surgery—against Miriam's wishes. I didn't want to admit it then, but the granddaughters had fallen victim to the typical, flawed view of paternalism: "doctor knows best." In this case, Dr. Roth knew more than Grandma did about what she wanted, what was good for her, and what she had planned. That, in hindsight, was just not empathetic.

Two days after her surgery, Miriam became lethargic and lost her capacity to speak. A repeat CT scan of the brain revealed a hemorrhage in the brain that occurred as a result of the surgery that I had performed.

I explained to the family that this was a most unfortunate complication. It would result in just what the patient stated she wanted to avoid: a loss of dignity. I was sorry and conveyed this to the granddaughters.

The family became undone. They felt betrayed. Ultimately, they sent me a letter that suggested that my motivation for doing the surgery was either based on naiveté or greed and they weren't sure which was worse.

I was devastated. Not only had I imposed my will on that of the patient, who had been clear about her desires, I had also incurred the hatred of her family. I felt foolish and vulnerable. I too had fallen victim to believing that because I felt strongly about something, my role was to talk the patient into seeing it through my lens. I had forgotten what paternalism was really all about—compassion, empathy, and seeing things first through the patients' eyes and meeting them where they are. Making a person feel irrelevant, implying that her age made her opinion not credible, going around her to consult relatives two generations younger than she, was not compassionate or empathetic at all. I basically ripped the Me right out of Medicine.

This was early in my career and I was yet to understand that such a horrible feeling would be an all too common part of my job. This is the nature of neurosurgery or is it? Certainly, uncertain outcomes are a part of any surgery—or anything for that matter—but imposing an opinion on someone, coaxing someone to my side, is nothing of the sort. In fact, that is not a narrative at all. It is hard enough to accept a bad result, but if I have been cavalier or not willing to give a case my best effort, a bad result becomes insufferable. In this case, imposing my will had the same result: devastation.

Who should decide what is the correct treatment for a patient? It is often posed as a conflict, pitting the doctor and the doctor-knows-best mentality (paternalism) against the patient and the patient-knows-herself-best mentality (patient autonomy). This dynamic has evolved over the past several decades with the pendulum swinging toward the patient.

Rather than view this dynamic as a conflict, I see an opportunity. Rather than thinking in terms of either-or, how about both? How about being practical about both roles and responsibilities the doctor and the patient have, and, especially, being more empathetic about the multifaceted and complex ways in which people see the world and make their decisions. All of our problems and all of our solutions rest in our perceptions of reality. Narrative-enhanced doctor paternalism plus narrative-enhanced patient autonomy can bridge the gap between the disparity of such perceptions and can result in a better doctor-patient relationship. If, as in any other relationship, we can effectively communicate "this is how I see it," and then form a decision based on the understanding that we either agree, agree to disagree, or land somewhere in the middle, patient autonomy can be instilled, while salvaging the empathetic paternalistic role of the doctor that has for generations been the epitome of medical practice. Ultimately, this optimal doctor-patient relationship is one of the promises of better medicine and begins first with doctors learning empathetic paternalism.

What Is Empathetic Paternalism?

Paternalism has come to be viewed in its simplest form as the belief both on the part of the patient *and the doctor* that the "doctor knows best." Envision the days of the old-fashioned doctor and his black leather bag, making house calls to sick patients. As he enters the home, a feeling of relief rolls through the family: "help is here." It wasn't just the clinical knowledge the family and patient expected to receive from the doctor, but the sense of deep compassion, genuine concern, and empathy, as no doubt, this doctor knew the dynamics of the family intimately, perhaps for the lifetimes of even its eldest members. Plus, this doctor has seen many things, many miracles and many defeats, and having someone to guide them during circumstances that have no context creates an aura of eminence.

Those days are gone. The compassion that goes hand-in-hand with a paternalistic nature is now vilified. It is no longer the compassionate doctor, but the self-serving one. Was I being compassionate toward Miriam's decision or empathetic as to what it might be like to be eighty-two and asked to take even the least chance of becoming what she might consider a "burden"? No.

But, treating paternalism as a black-and-white matter, either villain or hero, is not accurate either, and impedes the force that paternalism has on the practice of good medicine. After all, when we call someone "maternal," we say so with the utmost respect and honor, acknowledging that a woman has an instinct that compels her to put others before herself. Paternalism has the same meaning except it is applied to the opposite sex. If we can remember to see it that way, doctors would be less fearful to act paternalistically, while patients would be able to accept it for what it is—not a know-it-all, do-as-I-say message, but as one that is practical, wise, cooperative, and patient-first.

Ironically, squelching paternalism and placing patient autonomy above physician knowledge, experience, and guidance has not resulted in patient empowerment, but in a distrust of medicine. We have not only lost a wonderful conduit for compassion, but also another powerful feature of paternalism that is often overlooked—the capacity to affect change by introducing context.

What does this mean? Doctors are known to be great filters of information, but that doesn't mean that information is being translated properly to the patient. And if a self-proclaimed autonomous patient takes to the Internet solo, there is no further explanation of the information found. This is why doctors need to be listeners *and* storytellers. Long before people attended medical school, medicine men were ones who provided hope with treatment but also helped patients process information by providing context, inspiring hope, and instilling images that considered the perceptions the patient had. In this way, contextualization is highly personal and tailored to an individual. To boil it down further, doctors need to regain the skill of making information relatable, so the patient can make relative, and therefore, wiser decisions. This is why the greatest teachers have contextualized information through the creation of prolific, relatable parables, which are, in essence, the creation of narratives.

Because of this highly individualized and specialized contextualization of information, the empathetic paternalistic doctor has the power to change the patient and to even alter the disease or diagnosis. Just as the diagnosis of the disease has the capacity to change the patient (the chameleon effect), the doctor's capacity to contextualize the disease in a positive and constructive way also has the power to change the patient and, thus, the disease itself. Merriam-Webster defines contextualize as "to think about or provide information about the situation in which something happens."

This is what I did not do with Miriam. We did not engage in a narrative, the kind of dialogue that is necessary for an optimal give-and-take relationship. If I had, our discussion would have included an empathetic consideration of the perspective of an eighty-two-year-old. She had the right to decide what risks she was willing to take and to live with the natural history of her condition without surgery. I didn't fail the patient by being naïve or greedy, I failed by my lack of empathy. In the world where Me is put back into Medicine, the patient decides, but only after the doctor learns to understand and anticipate the complex and fascinating, sometimes deceitful, process we engage in when interpreting problems, weighting solutions, and living with our final decisions.

But that is only half the story. Patients ultimately need to come to terms with the factors that make the difference between good decision-making and bad decision-making and be conscious of what drives their decisions in the first place. In my opinion, patients who understand and accept what drives their conscious and subconscious biases, opinions, and desires are the most optimal examples of autonomy and are one of the most critical promises of putting back the Me in Medicine. As Pythagoras said, "No man is free who cannot command himself."

CHAPTER 7

The Promise of Better Decision-Making

"How are you feeling today?" I asked Elmer. Elmer, my patient, sat across from me in the office and had recently had a fusion operation on his lumbar spine. He was now about three months post-op. "I'm feeling pretty good," he replied. Pleased, I discussed a plan for the next couple of months and made my way to the next patient.

Later that day I became unsettled as I reviewed the latest data for my patient outcomes. Coincidentally, Elmer had also spoken with my nurse on the same day. In that setting, he suggested that he would not have undergone the surgery had he known before the surgery what he would feel like today.

I was struck by the disparity of the information that he gave to me and, on the same day, to the nurse. At first consideration, it would seem that the patient was generally unsatisfied, but felt uncomfortable conveying the information to his overbearing surgeon. But, that was not consistent with the relationship I had with Elmer. I am certain that he was being honest and that he felt comfortable telling me how he was feeling.

It turns out that both statements were true. Elmer was both happy and unhappy with the surgery.

We would like to believe that what we believe is what we really believe. We know that we can change our mind, but we attribute this to the dynamic consideration of new information *as* it becomes available. Even if we have a new belief, is it really a new belief? It turns out that it is more complicated than this. What we believe in a current place and time may be similar to the tip of an iceberg, where the bulk and core of that iceberg sits beneath our consciousness and is capable of holding more than one belief at the same time—even contradictory beliefs. In other words, we have the capacity to hold more than one belief in our subconscious state. What comes to the surface is often determined by current circumstances. This is the process by which we rationalize less than optimal outcomes. It is also an opportunity for the empathetic paternalistic doctor. I can partake in that selection of potential interpretations. This is the power of contextualization. As an empathetic paternalistic doctor, not only do I help the patient decide what to do, I also help the patient contextualize what has been done. In helping the patient select a positive spin on a result, I am actually affecting the outcome.

We have always thought of the objects around us as existing independently of us. There is a term, biocentrism, coined by Robert Lanza in 2007, which suggests conversely, that reality is best viewed as a brain's perception rather than something distinct outside of us. If a tree falls in the forest, does it make a sound? Most of us would find this age-old philosophical query a simple semantic issue and answer, "It depends on how you define sound." Biocentrism defines sound as distinctly and necessarily biological. Sound exists only in the brain and not "out there in nature." In fact, when a tree falls, it produces energy of many different frequencies of which only a small subset result in resonance of our hearing apparatus and are sound. In other words, energy needs a brain to become sound and sound doesn't exist otherwise.

This makes the brain a powerful organ and one of great influence over how we receive and interpret information. Reality is inexorably tied to our brains and can change depending on context.

Biocentrism and its underlying foundations in quantum mechanics, which also acknowledges that more than one reality can exist simultaneously, turns out to be quite similar to the idea of Elmer holding two seemingly disparate beliefs at the same time. Quantum mechanics suggests that human interaction collapses a spectrum of possible realities into one reality. In other words, we alter reality when we observe or measure it. Modern neuroscience teaches us that even our basic sensations such as sight and sound lie in a zone between fiction and non-fiction. We assume that what our eyes see is reality, but even our sensations are more of a virtual reality. Our brain takes some liberties as it puts its own spin on even our basic sensations. Similarly, our memories are not stored snapshots, but rather, editorialized, rationalized, and retro-fitted renditions of the past.

When Elmer is in different environments, he will allow different beliefs that he holds simultaneously to occupy his conscious state. He doesn't do this intentionally and there is nothing disingenuous about it. Understanding this has helped me remain empathetic when speaking with him and other patients. I now know that this is human nature and it underscores the import of my role as a doctor in drawing out the most appropriate beliefs. This is part of empathetic paternalism.

The important message here is that, as a doctor, I have the capability to help my patients, not only with the treatments rendered, but also with the ultimate interpretation of the results of those treatments. This represents the first limitation of decision-making. When anticipating possible outcomes, the patient must consider the possibility that both positive and negative outcomes will be altered over time by the way the patient contextualizes and rationalizes the results.

Heuristics

The problem with empathetic paternalism is that it takes time. But, in the office, I sense that patients want me to get to the point or tell them what to do rather than to develop an idea which is often a shade of gray and takes time to develop and understand. Patients are often afraid of ambiguity. This is due to the complexity of many decisions and a lack of confidence. This is not surprising as patients are forced to deal with a different vocabulary and a lack of understanding of human anatomy and physiology. They are tempted to simply let the doctor decide for them. This perpetuates a system that has been constructed to benefit the providers.

The promise comes when patients learn to abandon the concept of medicine as only a science and view it rather as a hermeneutical enterprise. Heuristics are mental shortcuts that we commonly utilize to help facilitate decision-making. Jerome Groopman has done a wonderful job of elucidating the processes that go through both the patient's and doctor's heads. Borrowing from the work of Daniel Kahneman, the psychologist who actually won a Nobel prize in economics for his work in explaining decision-making processes, Groopman outlines the use of heuristics to facilitate decision-making.

Part of becoming better patients who make better decisions is gaining an awareness of the heuristics that we use to facilitate our decisions. These heuristics are necessary as the decision processes in medicine are often extremely difficult to negotiate without a shortcut. Even though they are necessary, understanding their impact makes the patient a better decision maker.

The human brain is not capable of fully incorporating all of the potential variables of a proposed treatment when making a decision. If I tell a patient that the surgery is likely to help, but there is a less than 1 percent risk of death, that risk of death is impossible to weigh against the chance of success. Most patients simply ignore this risk similar in the way that we ignore the risk of a plane crashing when we choose to travel by air. In fact, when patients dwell on the improbable risks of a surgery, it tends to obscure the more important parts of the decision because the brain can only consider a limited number of variables at one time.

In surgery, the most common heuristic that I see is called availability bias. When I begin to lay out the pros and cons of a surgical procedure, the eyes of many of my patients often glaze over. Perhaps this is partially a result of how tediously I explain things, but mostly, patients find it hard because it *is* hard.

If a patient is asked to decide on an operation that has a 100 percent success rate and carries a 0 percent risk, the decision is relatively easy. Obviously, this is never the case. The patient has to weigh the risk of each potential complication against the proposed benefits of the surgery. This is something that we can't really do well. First, it is very difficult to imagine what each complication would feel like or what the proposed benefits would feel like. Second, it is hard to compare possibilities that occur over different time horizons. Is a reward offered now comparable to a potential side effect that occurs five years down the road? In addition, what the doctor and patient consider a success or a failure may differ. Finally, as discussed above, the outcome that the patient is considering is apt to change based on a natural process of contextualization that will invariably occur after the initial outcome.

The doctor may be able to approximate percentages of the various outcomes, but only the patient can determine the relative utility of each outcome. Utility takes into account not only the percentage of a particular outcome, but the personal import attached to that outcome. Daniel Bernoulli introduced this conceptual advance in the 1700s.

I commonly see this with my patients who are experiencing pain that has been refractory to treatment. If the surgery is to fail, some patients take comfort in knowing that they have done "everything possible" and thus even failure, in this setting, has a utility that the surgeon wouldn't necessarily anticipate.

Keeping track of so many variables is next to impossible and that is why patients turn to the shortcuts of heuristics. When I talk about a procedure and my patient's eyes glaze over, he is not calculating the relative utilities but rather, he is referencing a friend or family member who had a similar procedure and whether that person is happy with his or her decision. The procedure he references doesn't have to even be similar! Assuming that this is not the best way to make decisions, getting the patient to understand the heuristic he is utilizing can allow for a reconsideration and better process.

When Dante was deciding on whether to have a fusion for his back pain, he found the decision very difficult. His first instinct was to go for it. When I asked him why he felt this way, he told me that he had reached the end of his patience and he had faith in science. Finally, he had confidence in me as a surgeon. While these may be important, they have little to do with the pros and cons of the surgery that we were considering. They are all shortcuts that helped him make a decision. Knowing this, I needed to take the opportunity to open the dialogue further. Even if Dante said that he wants to go forward with the proposed surgery and feels "comfortable" with the decision, I need to force Dante to reflect on why he has made his decision. This is often a painful process for the patient because simply making a decision can serve as a relief and being pushed to acknowledge a dependence on shortcuts can restore the burden of uncertainty. But this process will end up in delivering a better ultimate decision.

A second common heuristic is the patient's proclivity for intervention. Most patients are on a spectrum between being naturalists or interventionists. Becoming a better decision-maker involves, in part, learning where on this spectrum one lies. For example, even though I am a surgeon, I sit well towards the naturalist end of this spectrum. This proclivity is based on my faith in the human body's capacity to heal itself naturally. It arises from the way that I was raised and from my earlier life experiences. I use this self-knowledge to guide me through choices of doing or not doing an intervention. In my case, I start off with the attitude that I will not have the procedure unless I am convinced that it makes sense, rather than the other way around. Other patients, like Dante, who believe in the power of science and medicine—after all, we put a man on the moon fifty years ago— tend to feel comfortable with an intervention and quickly accept the risks for the anticipated benefits. I often find myself talking such patients out of having surgery by having them examine their intervention-oriented proclivity.

When this spectrum was introduced to Dante, he recognized his interventionist temperament. This allowed him to step back and reconsider his options. He was able to consider a natural solution to his pain.

However, after several more minutes of discussion, he returned to opting for back surgery. This is an example of empathetic paternalism's capacity to address a patient's decision-making bias without compromising the patient's autonomy. The patient was rendered more capable so that he could make a better decision.

Decision-making is emotionally charged. George Loewenstein distinguishes between hot and cold emotional states in decision-making. The patient narrative helps tremendously with taking the patient out of the hot state. I often tell patients who are ready to sign up for surgery to go home and sleep on it. Sometimes they have a different opinion in the morning after they have cooled off.

Dante and I talked about the emotional component of his decision. He had been experiencing quite a bit of back pain in the days leading up to our discussion. He had found himself getting angry and emotional whenever the pain reared its head.

Dante, again, forced himself to step back and consider how much his emotional state was driving the decision. He promised to sleep on the decision and make it over the next couple of days rather than in the office while we were going over the choices.

Decision-making is facilitated, and thus undermined, by taking the easiest choice. This is another heuristic and happens frequently in medicine. If the doctor boldly asserts his opinion, acceptance is often easier than arguing. Related to this is our tendency to avoid the burden of the decision. Allowing the doctor to decide is often a relief. I often mention a bar scene analogy to my patients. If you are sitting in a bar and find someone across the bar attractive but feel tentative about walking over, you may ask your friend for advice. "Go for it" is what you will hear because it is an easy decision for your friend who doesn't feel the burden of the consequences. Similarly, you would likely tell your friend that he has nothing to lose. When you are deciding for yourself, it seems a lot harder.

Part of Dante wants me to tell him what to do. "You have seen so many patients like me," he said. "*You* tell me what to do." Part of me wants to tell him. It will save time. I have spent more time thinking about this decision and I have seen the results of many patients who have decided to do and not do surgery. Nonetheless, unlike my encounter with Miriam, my eighty-two-year-old brain tumor patient, I forced Dante to participate in this process. I know that if he relies on me and ends up less than satisfied, he will find the results harder to accept.

Decision-making is affected by anxiety and a lack of confidence in one's knowledge of a situation. This is humorously depicted by Peter Ubel as the "Ginger effect." When a patient is told they need surgery, the rest of the conversation is a blur of words that is obscured by the resounding echo of "surgery, surgery, surgery." Just as when Ginger (Ubel's dog) is reprimanded for getting into the garbage by a lecture from his owner on why such behavior is unhealthy and destructive, all the dog hears is, "blah blah, blah, Ginger, blah, blah, blah …"

In the world of fusion surgery, the Ginger effect is most often a deterrent. The word "surgery" or "fusion" is similar to "cancer" in that the other words in the sentence tend to fade away under the echo of the terrible buzzword. I have noticed that many patients simply shut down after they hear one of these words. This, too, limits the patient's capacity to make a good decision. I have to point this out to the patient. I often say, "I know you don't want surgery, but you have to listen to what it entails in order to make an informed decision." This redirection is very helpful to patients. Even those who reject surgery are ultimately happy that they spend the time deeply thinking when considering surgery.

Deep Thinking

Education has been shown to be an independent determinant of health. Wealthy patients enjoy better health. This is not because they can afford better doctors or medications, but because they are more likely to learn and become a participant in the decision-making process. In the future, The Internet will increasingly be the source for patients to learn about medicine. The majority of people already routinely turn to the Internet to research their health issues.

Surfing the Internet is like navigating the Wild West. There is an abundance of uncensored and misleading information. It is difficult to sort out what is educational from what is an advertisement. There is an abundance of information, which is a great thing, but its abundance can be a source of frustration.

Earlier I talked about being a young doctor; despite all that I had learned in medical school, I was struggling to make even simple decisions about patient care. I looked at this as the difference between knowledge and wisdom. While the former is relatively easy to acquire, the latter requires an extra effort or a process of shaping or reprocessing the knowledge.

The Internet epitomizes the abundance of knowledge. Surfing the Internet exposes us to an endless array of numerically labeled shortcuts to knowledge—the numbers are seductive: "7 reasons to . . ., 5 ways of . . .," etc. These bursts of knowledge are dangerous. Not because they are false, but because they effortlessly provide knowledge where wisdom is needed. They also provide immense satisfaction making them all the more dangerous. The number attached to an Internet article is particularly enticing, as the reader knows up front that the effort to learn will be limited to that number. This is particularly intoxicating in our quick-fix society. The majority of people browse the Internet for pleasure. There is a literal dopamine surge (the pleasure hormone) when we get on the Net. Surfers are also junkies for information. While this is better than passive surfing for pleasure, it is still not enough. What I am calling for is an even more intense form of reading—reading to learn and acquire wisdom rather than knowledge.

There is a symbiotic process between a writer and a reader. There is a cross pollination of ideas. The reader gets into the writer's head and, as such, is transformed. This is an active and deliberate process where imagination, empathy, and cognitive processes are in full throttle. Perhaps the surfing of the Internet can release dopamine and pleasure with its spurts of knowledge, but the process of deep thinking and learning delivers a greater and more sustained release of dopamine.

I read everything twice because it is often in the second reading that a "meeting of the minds" occurs. It is better to sacrifice breadth in our reading than depth. Part of reading is staying with the author the whole way through. The presence of hyperlinks on the Internet, while allowing invaluable explorations into what the reader wants to pursue, also prevent the reader from being forced to finish the task. It is in finishing the task that the transformation often occurs. Because the writer understands that our attention spans are diminishing, he or she feels obligated to get to the point earlier and does not fully develop the argument.

In the office, I sense that patients want me to get to the point or tell them what to do rather than to develop an idea which is often a shade of gray and takes time to develop and understand. Patients are often afraid of ambiguity. In order to be an active participant in the narrative and be better and more confident decision-makers, patients need to learn some of the vocabulary and science, and most of all, how to interpret statistics. Doctors need to more fairly introduce such information, contextualize it, and lead the patient to pursue wisdom over knowledge.

Numeracy

The deep thinking and self-education required to make good decisions would be severely impeded if a person were illiterate. As with the inability to read words, the inability to understand numbers, known as innumeracy, also negatively affects the ability to make weighty decisions. Just as narrative medicine requires literacy on behalf of patients, it requires people have numeracy.

To enter medical school, all students have to demonstrate proficiency in calculus. As a physics major, I found calculus invaluable as a tool to understand many phenomena, but not in the realms of medicine. Statistics, which is not a required course, forms the basis of understanding risk in medicine, which ends up being part of almost all decisions. When doctors (or patients) try to understand the medical literature, statistics are also vital. Studies often show trends that are not statistically significant. What are the chances that the study's findings could be the result of chance alone? Becoming a doctor and becoming a patient is greatly enhanced by a general understanding of statistics. Statistics conceptually underlie all decisions.

The future of medicine will increasingly depend on our use of statistics. As medicine transitions from fee-for-service to fee-for-value, we will need to better understand how we define and prove value. This will be impossible without understanding statistics.

Managing risk also requires some sophistication of statistics. Suppose I tell a forty-year-old patient that the risk of his aneurysm rupturing is 2 percent per year and that the risk of serious morbidity with the treatment of the aneurysm is 5 percent. The patient has to compare the cumulative risk of 2 percent per year over his projected lifetime with the 5 percent risk of having surgery today. This is really tough to do. How do I manage this as his surgeon? Do I simply tell him that the statistics have been "worked out" and intervention has been shown to be statistically indicated? In this setting, the patient need not think, but simply trust and sign on the dotted line. Conversely, do I educate him on the process? The chances are that he has some degree of innumeracy and that he cannot intuitively calculate the risk of rupture over the next ten years. Many patients who hear that there is a 2 percent risk of hemorrhage per year assume that this presents a 20 percent risk over ten years and a 40 percent risk over twenty years, and so on. Obviously, extending this logic to fifty years suggests that the aneurysm would have greater than 100 percent chance of rupturing.

But, the way to look at risk in this setting over a number of years is to look at the rate of *not* rupturing. There is a 98 percent chance of not rupturing over the next year and a $.98 \times .98 = 96$ percent chance of not rupturing over two years, etc. This is a comparison that is not so easy for a human mind to perform.

The narrative thus becomes essential in any discussion of statistics. The doctor must be reasonably well-versed in statistics to provide the narrative. A rudimentary knowledge attained by the patient is also essential. Numeracy is yet another path by which doctors can become better doctors and patients better patients and where decisions are made optimally. Once the patient with an enraptured aneurysm, that taking into account his age and the risk of the procedure, understands that statistically surgery is a good idea, the decision-making process becomes significantly easier.

When Emma and I discussed the success rate of surgery, she was initially fixated on hearing what number I would produce. As I felt the need to qualify my ultimate answer, I started to explain to her how I came up with the number, but Emma jumped in, saying, "Just give me the number!" The problem is that I cannot give a number of a projected success without first defining success. How do I know that Emma and I share the same definition? I told Emma that I define success, not as being pain-free—which is an unrealistic expectation from her type of surgery—but rather, as being very happy with her decision to do surgery when asked about the surgery at three months, six months, and twelve months post-op. It is much easier for the patient to focus on success only after both the patient and the doctor are talking about the same things.

If you remember our previous discussions about human nature and its capacity to rationalize outcomes, you will realize that some patients have the capacity to spin a positive light on a less-than-ideal outcome while others can do the exact opposite, spin a negative light on what is a reasonable outcome. This ability to change perspective makes the "success rate" much harder to predict.

In fact, any success rate that I give to my patients is, at best, a rough guess and should be presented as such. Dr. Yuan, an old and wise neurosurgeon and mentor of mine, once reminded me that the burden is not on me to supply a number, because that number is impossible to accurately devise. The burden is on the patient who has to decide. That decision is both difficult to do and will undoubtedly be biased by the use of heuristics, emotional states, and other irrational factors. I do have a burden in this process and that burden is what creates the promise of better decision-making, because it means I acknowledge that I must serve as a shepherd for the patient—one who has the humility and empathy to listen, as well as teach. Ultimately the promise is an empowered relationship that allows for shared decision-making and improved decisions.

Healthy Skepticism of the Science of Medicine

When a patient sits in the doctor's office and is given some recommendations by the doctor, it is difficult to know whether the recommendations are based on "gut" feelings, anecdotal experience, or science. Often the recommendations are based on some combination of the three. There are also some other factors that come into play. Many of the doctor's recommendations are related to habit—the way the doctor has managed a problem for years. This has some merit, but there are some doctors that do things the same way for decades, and in that case, habit may represent something that is no longer optimal. Even more dangerous than not changing is changing simply because something newer (and presumed better) has come along. Or worse, a change that was prompted by an attractive or charismatic salesman. Much has been written about the capacity for the pharmaceutical industry to affect behavior through advertising either to doctors or directly to patients. This is easy to criticize but persists despite our knowledge and rebuke of its practice.

The theme of this chapter is to learn to identify certain factors that affect our decision-making. The last important one that patients and doctors need to incorporate when faced with discussing challenges and solutions is a healthy skepticism of the science of medicine.

Asking oneself, *"How strong is the science that guides the doctor's recommendations?"* can go a long way in forming a more educated opinion while avoiding mental shortcuts. In fact, this kind of healthy skepticism is strengthened by the other practices previously discussed, such as developing numeracy and being aware of biocentrism.

There has been a push for doctors to make recommendations by relying on evidence-based medicine. The idea that a recommendation is made on the basis of "that's how I've been doing it" has humorously been dubbed "eminence-based" medicine. It's funny until we acknowledge how frequently this occurs.

What about evidence-based medicine? This concept demands that decisions are not made by tradition, habit, or influence from advertising. The decisions should be derived from the accumulated literature. Unfortunately, that literature is not all equally helpful and terribly incomplete. For example, a study done prospectively and randomized with controls that are not treated or even controls that are treated with placebo is typically more meaningful than a study that retrospectively looks at the same topic. There are processes of meta-analysis where the accumulated literature is examined for solid conclusions after the individual studies are weighted.

The problem is, although the literature is vast, it provides surprisingly few solid recommendations. Also, these recommendations often apply to a disease in general, but not necessarily to a particular individual with the disease. The more individualized we require our evidence-based medicine to be, the harder it is to find the data. Each study is time-consuming and expensive. The funding often comes from the very companies that would benefit from a positive result making the conclusions suspect.

The future science of medicine will benefit from the rising accumulation and sharing of data. Each participating patient will need to share his or her data. Obviously, the information will need to be shared in such a way as to not violate the individual patient's privacy. But the data of the future will be vast and the technology will be sufficiently powerful to manage and manipulate it in ways to help us better decide what to do in a given situation.

Traditionally, medicine has progressed in a way that would surprise many patients. Typically, ideas will arise through inference, logic, or even fortuitous observation. They are postulated and then left to be disproved. This sequence of events was brought to light by Karl Popper. This is not to say that the method is a bad one, but understanding this sequence demands that patients view "standards of care" more critically. At times these "yet to be disproved" ideas are viewed as proven. They become recommendations of doctors. Only years later are they disproven, or worse, proven to be detrimental. Listening to what is the "new" treatment needs to be carefully considered rather than rapidly adapted.

With this excess of information there will be opportunity, but who is going to tend to the information? The data, in total, will be a source of discovery and progress, but each individual's data will need to be tended to, interpreted, and used as a source of personal change. This cannot be subjugated to the doctor. Yes, the doctor will be essential to provide the fine details of education and the contextualization. But in the end, it must be digested and managed by the patient, who has become acutely aware of what threatens or inspires his or her decision-making and is autonomous as a result.

CHAPTER 8

The Promise of the Autonomous Patient

An ancient Indian parable speaks of a man with bare feet who wants to walk across a field of thorns and has two options: he can pave a path in the field, or he can make himself sandals. In the former case, he sets out to change what is around him, while in the latter case, he chooses to change himself. Autonomy is a responsibility to oneself. Now that we understand how we create an autonomous mindset, we can focus on the importance of exercising it, fortifying it, and preserving it. Autonomy does not mean "acting alone." It is to self-govern and be independent and confident enough to work harmoniously and successfully *alongside* a doctor.

The concept of being an autonomous patient and a good decision maker has traditionally included being conscientious with medications, going for regular checkups, and keeping one's blood pressure and cholesterol regulated. While I don't disagree with these ideas in principle, I worry that they are dangerous. Not because they are wrong but because may serve as a distraction.

Autonomy commonly plays out like this: "I haven't been to the doctor in a while. I should get a checkup." This stems from the underlying idea that we often suspect or worry that there is some bad process brewing inside of us, undetected, but potentially discoverable. If we could just expose it, we would catch it early and treat it more effectively. Autonomy is thus seen as initiating an action.

We naively think that going for a checkup will suffice, or better yet, we hope for a negative checkup, which will give us peace of mind. But what is a checkup? We get a stethoscope placed over our hearts, our abdomens palpated, labs drawn, and most importantly, we are asked a series of questions that may tip off our experienced doctor that something is wrong. We are hoping that the encounter will be meaningful.

Better yet would be a whole body scan. Why not look for everything possible while we are healthy so that we can detect and more effectively treat whatever we find? This can be done. For a generous fee—not covered by insurance—one can have his or her whole body scanned and scrutinized.

The problem here is that screening for improbable things ends up uncovering incidental findings that create more questions or the need for biopsies. Findings that are not treatable can carry an emotional burden, another risk of indiscriminate screening.

A poorly understood corollary of statistics reveals that when screening for improbable entities, we uncover more false positives than true positives. In other words, what is revealed in the test is more likely not real than real, and yet, we are stuck with the positive and the plenty of follow up tests and anxiety that follows.

The promise is that the checkup of the future is going to be different. Rather than a cursory exam and conversation that may or may not be fruitful, there will be value in the checkup of the future. Part of that value will come from technology and part will come from narrative medicine.

Technology is ushering in what has being called an "omic" revolution. The name omic comes originally from genomics, which is the idea of sequencing our genes in order to get a blueprint of how our life will unfold. Having one's genome sequenced has become progressively less expensive. As data is accrued, it will also become progressively more useful. Eventually, it will become a routine part of our medical records.

The Omics Revolution

The project of sequencing the genome was extraordinary and stands as one of science's greatest accomplishments, but the idea that we can make meaningful forecasts based solely on our genetic blueprint has proved to be quixotic.

Despair not, however, because we also have epigenetics. Epigenetics is the link between our genome and our environment. It is a new way of looking at the age-old debate between nature and nurture. In fact, there should no longer be a debate—it is always nature *and* nurture and never nature or nurture because nurture can change nature.

Epigenetics involves modifications of the genome through production of an RNA (ribonucleic acid) that can select parts of the DNA to be activated and alter the three-dimensional shape of the RNA based on environmental changes.

We have always known that our bodies can change based on what we choose to do (e.g., exercise), but we only are now understanding that those changes also occur in our genomic blueprint as well as in our appearance.

The human genome is huge compared with genomes of other animals, but the extra DNA doesn't just code our proteins, cell body structure, and capacity to reproduce. It is an extraordinarily complicated piece of information that allows our individual cells to adapt to a changing and variable environment by turning on or off or altering our DNA. How could it be otherwise? No design of information could ever anticipate an arbitrary environment. The design would have to incorporate a method of adaptation.

In addition to genomics and epigenomics, several other omics have been explained and can be added to the potential future of medicine as it relates to creating more patient autonomy and self-awareness.

Proteomics (the study of proteins) suggests that a blood test done in the office can sample the array of proteins active in the blood as an indicator of real-time health. In other words, we can assess current health through looking at the thousands of active proteins.

Metabolomics (the study of chemical processes), similarly, looks at our blood for the real time chemical processes that leave a footprint of the thousands of cellular reactions taking place.

Exposomics is a quantified list of our exposure to environmental toxins such as heavy metals, radiation, etc. It is a synopsis of what we have been subjected to in our environment.

Finally, **microbiomics** is the aspect of our health attributable to the billions of bacteria and that live on and within us. This is a nascent field in medicine that is sure to grow and help us understand our current health.

In addition to the omics revolution, our activities, vital signs, and many other medical attributes will be increasingly quantifiable. This will occur as the result of medical sensors, which will soon be a standard part of our smartphone functions. Phone-based sensors are inexpensive and rapidly proliferating in scope and are manage autonomously by the patient. The acquired data will be fodder for the wave of big data that will become part of our health profile. This data will be owned and managed by each of us.

Tomorrow's Checkup

Let's imagine now how the checkup of the future will look. Our medical record will include our genome. This will provide a basic template on how we should live. We will understand many of our potential vulnerabilities and strengths and develop individualized life plans designed to maximize our health.

We will come to the office with a downloaded synopsis of our activity. Rather than answer the meaningless question "Have you been active?" with the equally meaningless, "Moderately," patients' own accelerometers, step counters, and other sensors on their smartphones will provide an exact, quantified answer. There is no reason to take a blood pressure measurement in the office when your blood pressure over the past three months is already available.

Once in the office (or maybe even at home) we will have a small sample of body fluid checked for the active proteins and metabolites. Microbiomes and exposomes will be similarly quantifiable. Now patient will be able to sit down with their doctor with a true account of their current health.

The utility of the office visit of the future will not be in an unveiling of this sacred data, for the data will be democratized and already *owned by the patient*. The utility will be in the educational, contextual, and strategic synergy that will arise from the doctor-patient relationship as the data are considered.

There is great power to be had on the part of the autonomous patient, but with great power comes great responsibility, without which, patients will impede the promise of the Me in Medicine.

Agency

It has been demonstrated that when cardiologists tell their patients that they must change their lifestyle or they will die from their cardiac disease, only a small percentage of people will actually change. Even though these patients understand the danger that they are in and sincerely want to make changes, most are unable to affect the necessary change. Why is this?

If you were given a ridiculous pill that claimed to prolong your life, each day that passed would add personal conviction to its false claim. Even if you understood that the claims were not founded in science, would you be hesitant to stop taking the pill? Breaking habits takes courage and often goes against the grain. It is often easier to persist in our habits even when we know they make no sense. Courage is needed because we have something called loss aversion.

Most people will not enter a coin toss bet where they stand to win 100 dollars with heads and lose 100 dollars with tails. This is not too surprising, but what may be surprising is that heads has to yield close to 200 dollars versus the 100 dollars for tails for people to take the bet. This is an example of loss aversion. Loss aversion promotes a status quo philosophy. If you are on a medication for a long time and you learn that the drug is not proven beneficial, do you continue on the drug? Chances are that the answer is yes because stopping the med risks losing something.

Agency is a social science term and is defined as the capacity of individuals to act independently and to make their own free choices. Being dictated by fear and loss aversion impedes free will. Without agency, we have no autonomy. In order to preserve and utilize our autonomous mindset, we need to incite agency.

Agency is lost because we are distracted from action. In Part I: The Problem, we discussed technology's tendency to distract us. It is helpful to view our free time as a battle between agency and distraction. With the proliferation of technology, our capacity to maintain the "task at hand" has suffered a lethal blow. Business interests have learned to engage this vulnerability and leverage our distractibility to influence us. The more we live in the cyber world, the more susceptible we will be to the interests of others. Agency requires deliberate time and focus to be sustainable. The key to agency is deliberately taking the time to formulate a plan. Agency is essential in being an autonomous patient.

There are online games, access to a near infinite amount of new and exciting information, emails to answer, etc. There is no doubt that some of us get lost in this cyber world and do so at the expense of some of our goals. It is the more subtle loss of agency that I am interested in, however, and how it pertains to healthcare.

The most common loss of agency that I see is in the avoidant patient who worries about a behavior, but deals with it by pretending that it doesn't exist or by developing techniques to avoid thinking about it. This is typical of the smoker who is quick to say, "I really should stop." This phrase is repeated abstractedly as an acknowledgment of the dangers of smoking and as an avoidance of conflict, and is designed to last until the subject is mercifully changed. By being agreeable, the patient is being avoidant. The bottom line: nothing changes.

Another variant of this avoidance is the habit of self-labeling and the subsequent hiding behind that label. This is seen in the overweight patient who believes and states incessantly that he has no discipline. Each time he is faced with the choice of food selection, the self-proclaimed label serves as an excuse for the choice. The bottom line: nothing changes.

More subtle, is the patient who seemingly confronts a problem, but selects as a target, not the whole problem but a part of the problem that is easy to address. This is part of the bait-and-switch mentality discussed earlier. We use it all of the time when trying to make decisions. We substitute something easier to focus on when we decide that we must take some action because it is easier. A classic example of this is the patient with heart disease who focuses on the treatment of cholesterol. By picking a surrogate target (cholesterol) rather than the important subject of cardiac health, the patient feels like he is exercising agency, but falls short on accepting the full burden of agency.

4P Medicine

The burden of agency can be accepted by anticipating the future of medicine, the new responsibilities of its players, and the different roles and expectations doctors and patients will assume. Just as this book has been divided into four parts, all represented by P's—Problem, Promise, Philosophy, and Prescription—the future of healthcare has similarly been described as 4P Medicine, a term coined by the biologist Leroy Hood. It refers to medicine of the future, which he predicts will be predictive, preventative, personalized, and participatory. Autonomous patients will be synonymous with the ability to understand and implement these traits in order to optimize healthcare.

Predictive

Most of our ability to predict will arise from the rapidly accumulating databases derived from having our genomes sequenced. The other omics discussed previously will provide more real time data as well.

Predictive medicine will need to protect privacy and promote optimism. Sequencing the genome will invariably lead to an uncovering of vulnerabilities. As doctors, we must not let this affect our population's insurability. The vulnerabilities can also undermine our confidence. I believe that we will adapt by embracing the power of epigenetics. We will find ways to alter our genome or marginalize our vulnerabilities through how we live. Currently we all know that we are going to die, but most of us don't dwell on this reality. We construct our lives in a state of suspended disbelief. We will take the same approach if we discover that we are susceptible to a particular disease process.

Preventive

An ounce of prevention is worth a pound of cure. Preventive medicine would seem a no-brainer.

One of the rationales for mandating healthcare is to provide the opportunity to prevent disease, or at least, manage disease, rather than treat those already floridly ill in an emergency room setting. The presumption is that those with access to healthcare will better tend to their health. The government already mandates vaccines and seatbelts, which are examples of preventive medicine.

One of the opportunities of preventive medicine is in screening. The use of screening presumes that it will be beneficial to those screened. This is not always easy to determine, however. The hidden problem with screening is that it ends up as a vehicle for more treatment. This has been explored in chapter 4.

Screening for cancer presents another issue. Some of the cancers discovered aren't necessarily more treatable when found early. Others don't always need treatment. In these settings, screening doesn't make sense as the diagnosis offers little upside and the further testing and angst discussed above bring about a real downside.

In summary, predictive medicine will create opportunities for preventive medicine. Demonstrating utility in our preventions and not merely assuming their worth will best serve us.

Personalized

Personalized medicine is not new. We have eyeglasses, dentures, and prostheses. Personalized medicine of the future will be more powerful. We will be able to predict individual responses from specific medications and treatments. This has been called pharmacogenomics. This transformation is already on the way in the use of chemotherapy. Personalized medicine will allow us to know, when taking a medication with a 10 percent response rate, which 10 percent will respond. This is a critically important piece of information. Back pain is potentially amenable to personalized medicine. We know that no single treatment is predictably useful for acute back pain, but if subdivided and personalized, specific types of back pain in individual patients, may be more predictably helped.

Participatory

Patient involvement is one of the main themes of this book. As patients participate more, they will alter the construct of medicine and benefit more. Success in the treatment of back pain demands patient autonomy and patient self-efficacy. Earlier I discussed the flooding of data that biological sensors will provide. This information must be owned and interpreted by patients.

What patients often fail to realize is that even a great doctor who is empathetic, knowledgeable, and motivated will need to focus on the next patient once the current patient leaves. Based on time limitations and demands, doctors end up being reactive more than proactive. The patient must be his own advocate and not assume that someone else is looking after him. The patient must try to learn some of the necessary medical language and physiological concepts of his disease process. Education is the single most important enabler of health and this requires patient participation. The promise of technology can help bring these necessities to the forefront.

CHAPTER 9

The Promise of Technology

The Internet is a double-edged sword. It is both a source of information and a distracting substitute for real learning. The key is how we approach it. Being the recipient of a near infinite display of novel information is addictive. Addictions can be hard to break. Surfing puts us in the mode of "liking what we see." The purpose of learning is the opposite. It allows for "seeing what we like."

To illustrate this point, let's consider shopping for a book. There is nothing wrong with liking what we see. It is thrilling to walk about Barnes and Noble and enjoy the displays. Not infrequently, we find a book that seems perfect. It may be a book that we would never have considered except for the taste of an arbitrary encounter with a display chosen by another person. Sometimes fortuitous events pay off more than those carefully planned.

This passive approach to culture, media, and the arts will suit our exploratory nature and fill in our deficiencies. It is both impractical and unpredictable, however. It is not the way to approach medicine.

The Internet has made possible a different method to explore information. This method is active rather than passive and may add to our strengths and interests. It is planned and predictable. It is seeing what we like and it is ideal for patient autonomy.

Let's use music as an analogy. Growing up I listened to whatever the radio station DJs decided to play (which was controlled by the big music labels). I would like a small percentage of what I heard and my collection of music progressed slowly. Contrast that method to one that I use today. It accrues songs based on structural similarities or on recommendations from listeners with similar sensibilities. In this setting, the chance of liking what I hear is increased significantly and my collection can expand quickly.

We all have a personal taste in music and the question is whether it is better to add to what we like or to be exposed to different sounds and to broaden out horizons.

In other words, do we strive for depth or breadth?

In culture and arts, a combination of depth and breadth is essential. In medicine, depth should trump breadth. Depth is essential because if patients are passive or superficial in their pursuit, they will continue to be victimized by the system.

The way to approach the Internet is like a researcher writing a paper. The reader should have a specific topic in mind. He should seek comprehensive articles on the subject and read the entire article. The Internet should be treated like a book. Once there is a basic understanding, the reader can branch out and read either more specific or complicated pieces or even access the original studies.

This is not currently readily available. There are often exorbitant charges to read articles. It is hard for even experienced readers to recognize what is substantiated information, what is anecdotal information, and what is fabricated or merely advertisement.

Earlier in the book I discussed the need for doctors to contribute their narratives regarding the aspects of patient care for which they consider themselves experts. This will be an invaluable source for patients to understand the application of what they have learned—to convert knowledge into wisdom. It will also serve as a modern referral method. Doctors have been hesitant to advertise, as it often feels cheap to us. The Internet allows doctors to share content. Having an online platform, which is available and transparent to the patient, will prove to be much better than the traditional referral practice.

In medicine today, doctors often refer to their friends or to those that will refer back. Referrals tend to change very slowly as doctors practice in their own silos and fail to keep abreast of what is changing around them. This is not ideal for patients. The autonomous patient of the future will manage his own referrals by accessing the doctor's online platform from a search on the Internet. This will serve doctors well as they will be able to self-promote by simply providing content. In today's world, content is at the core of advertising. Patients will base their choice on their perusal of the Internet rather than on the old-fashioned referral methods.

The Internet will also allow information to flow among patients who experience similar symptoms. New information has traditionally disseminated slowly. Access for the patient required waiting to see the doctor with the hope that he was privy to something new and better. The democratization of information will put the information directly in the patient's hands. It will frequently be the vested patient telling the doctor what is new and better.

Chat rooms will allow patients with similar health issues to exchange ideas about coping with disease, toxicities of treatment, and quality of doctors. Diagnostic mysteries can be posted online to allow the cumulative experience of many different doctors to submit their intuition or input. How many times have you had a problem solved by someone who just happened to know a lot about your particular problem? It is seemingly effortless and you can't help but feel lucky that you have happened upon this person. In medicine, we have the potential to make this less a matter of luck by posting the circumstances of a particular problem online and letting many experts look at the problem. In this respect, the Internet becomes a diagnostic amplifier. This will greatly increase the chance of someone identifying a great solution based on his unique experience.

For doctors, this is both a little threatening and a little exciting, as it will force us to raise our game. The more that information is democratized, the more up to date we have to be.

In general, transparency is always both threatening and exhilarating. The doctor must be a curator of information. Our narratives should be transparently accessible to patients on the Internet. As a surgeon, the patient should have access to how often I perform a particular procedure. The patient should also have access to my interpretation of the science and practice of medicine. Edith Wharton said, "There are two ways of spreading light: to be the candle or the mirror that reflects it." This is a great way of considering how we can function as curators. Not all of us can be candles but even if we merely reflect the light, we are spreading information and allowing for resonance.

The Department of Health is executing a strategic plan for the coming years to dramatically expand health information technology. In this initiative, the information in individual offices and hospitals will be universally available and communicative. This will connect all of our patient encounters. It will commoditize the traditional office and hospital visit. Computers will begin to replace many of our tasks. The increased information will allow for improved understanding of our disease processes and for increased evidence for individualized treatments. This will occur as super-computers will analyze the surplus of data and uncover correlations. Correlations have been one of the main drivers of medical progress. It has often been pointed out that correlations are not causations. We tend to overrate correlations and introduce new treatments based on correlations—before we have proven causation. These ideas are often reversed when better evidence-based medicine refutes their efficacy. Big data of the future will have the capability of generating more accurate correlations once the majority of our experiences are connected. All of this is great, as long as we don't let our technological advances detract from our humanity.

The Internet can also act as a memory enhancer. Human memory is a complex process. A part of our deep temporal lobes called the hippocampus acts like a conductor and holds memory for a period of time. It orchestrates the relationships of the memory to various sensory systems (visual, auditory, olfactory, etc.) and modifies the memory in accordance with these many sensory cortex areas. It is in this way that memory is creatively built, rather than transcribed like a photo from a negative. Seneca's version of memory is the incorporation of what has been learned into a personal context; it is a creation—something unique—of the subject's personal experience and previous learning. The Internet can serve as an alternative or surrogate memory holder that allows for a more objective account or reality. It can free the mind up for the process of deep thinking. Isn't it better to have all of your contacts' phone numbers on your phone so you can use your brainpower for something more meaningful? Einstein described education as that which is left behind when all that was learned in school has been forgotten. We don't even have to worry about forgetting now. Having all this information readily available allows us to learn less. Learning less, in this light, is an advantage, as it frees our brains for thinking.

There is no doubt that as we use a new technology, it not only empowers us, but it also changes us. The part of the brain that corresponds to the left hand of a violin player becomes different—it becomes overdeveloped. Similarly, the brain of a deep learner will certainly become different than that of an Internet surfer.

Technological Ownership

The patient of the future will own his own medical records. They will all be at his fingertips—literally—on his laptop and on his smartphone. It will be like an online brokerage account where one can track one's finances.

As we continue to take in unprecedented amounts of data, and use the data in an unprecedented way now that the computing power is available, we will understand more and more the relationship between our health and what we can do to attain more health. The data will come in effortlessly through sensors. Having this displayed in real time will end up being a strong motivating factor and make it easier to take responsibility for our health. Technology has brought us the smartphone and with it the capability to connect to the Internet anytime and anywhere. Chris Anderson, author of *The Long Tail: Why the Future of Business is Selling Less of More,* says that we are now children of the petabyte age. Kilobytes were stored on floppy discs. Megabytes were stored on hard discs. Terabytes were stored on disc arrays. Petabytes are stored in the cloud. This exponential access to data is part of the new medicine. What will be transformative to medicine, however, is the proliferation of biological sensors. These are relatively inexpensive, wearable, and connectable sensors that will produce enormous amounts of data. There will be sensors for our heart, our blood, and our brain. There will be sensors to monitor what we have eaten, how much activity we have done and how much sleep we have gotten. Analysis and interpretation of this data will, in turn, have the capacity to transform medicine by introducing and refining numerous correlations. It is essential that patients own this data and use it to promote health. If these data belong to the medical system, it will be used to justify more unnecessary diagnoses and treatments.

CHAPTER 10

The Promise of the Placebo

While technology is undeniably changing the face of health-care, we cannot dismiss the power of the human body and its ability to heal itself. Medicine has a long history of taking credit for what should more appropriately be attributed to the awe-in-spiring design of the human body. Much of what substantiated old systems of thought was that interventions based on these theories were seen to lead to improvement of patients. But those improve-ments were in spite of, rather than because of, the interventions.

The accomplishments of doctors have historically parasitized off of the natural adaptability of the body to heal itself. Despite the proliferation of effective treatments over the past century, doctors continue to take credit for the highly adaptable bodies that they tend to.

Many medications can also be thought of as parasites. Pain medication works by tapping into our endogenous systems of pain control. Have you ever stopped to consider why we have receptors for opiates in our bodies? It is because we have our own "natural" painkillers that opiates fortuitously parasitize off of.

Much has been written about the placebo effect. The very root of the word placebo is from ancient priests "faking" emotions at funerals. But what if we look at the placebo effect as any inter-vention that taps into our body's natural capacity to adapt to its environment? If we take a sugar pill and derive pain control from the pill when we are told that it is a painkiller, it is the suggestion that ignites our natural pain stifling mechanisms. Is that any more "fake" than taking an opiate that parasitizes off the very same mechanism? In fact, when we incite our endogenous pain stifling mechanisms, our breathing and heart rate slow—just as if we have ingested an opiate.

You see, much of the positive affect that medicine has had over the centuries is likely a placebo effect. It should not be marginalized but embraced and placed next to the other medical and technological advances made in medical care.

There is a flip side as well. Some of our disease processes are attributable to the placebo effect's evil stepsister, the nocebo effect. The nocebo effect is the capacity of the brain to ignite processes that undermine our well-being. Diseases such as fibromyalgia, irritable bowel syndrome, and chronic fatigue disease may ultimately be more usefully conceptualized as the result of the nocebo effect. This thinking does not minimize their significance, but allows for different approaches of treatment. If the brain is capable of resetting our pain threshold or energy stores, working on our brain rather than eliminating pain or increasing energy may prove to be a more fruitful approach.

The splitting of diseases into silos of organic or psychological etiology has long been a tradition in medicine. Perhaps it is a residual mindset of the mind-body distinctions set forth by René Descartes in the 17th century. Rather than looking at the mind-body as an either-or, if we embrace the synergy of the mind and body as both a source of our illness and a source of our healing, we allow for the powers of empathetic paternalism and patient autonomy to emerge as sources of health.

This may seem disingenuous or less than fully scientific, but modern neuroscience teaches us that we are not passive receptors of information, but we create our information. Even our basic sensations such as sight and sound are, in part, virtual reality. The brain takes some liberties as it puts its own spin on even our basic sensations. What we see, hear, and feel depend on what we expect, what we have previously experienced, and on our cultural upbringing.

Disease and health should be similarly considered. We experience health and disease, but we also create disease and health. Earlier, we discussed epigenetics and the role that our environment plays on the expression of our genomes. Our minds also have an impact on our genomes through epigenetics. This helps to explain "blue zones," which are areas in the world with improved longevity that appears to arise not only from better health habits, but also, social connectedness—the mind's epigenetic influence. We create health and disease through our interpretations of what we feel and through epigenetic expression of our genomes. We should embrace the extraordinary technology and science of medicine, but simultaneously recognize the power of our minds over our bodies. We should consider the scientific basis of disease, but also look at the placebo and nocebo effects as a spectrum of the mind's involvement and control of our health.

Much of medicine's success in the past can be retrospectively evaluated as due to the compassionate doctor's contextual influence rather than the treatments rendered. We now know that those treatments were worthless, but when rendered, the patients believed in their efficacy.

While seemingly demoting the importance of our beliefs by characterizing them as malleable, it also allows for a potential positive consequence. The interactions with my patients not only serve to diagnose, teach, and comfort, but can partake in how my patients actually feel.

The placebo effect not only ignites natural processes in the body but it also affects how we feel about what is happening in our bodies. It gets back to the important distinction between what is wrong and how we feel. We can change how we feel, and, to an extent, by doing such, change what is actually wrong.

If we view the world of back pain from this perspective, we may get a better understanding of why our current treatments have failed. Many of the current paradigms involve identifying the elusive pain generator and fixing it. When this is not possible (the majority of the time), we turn to treating the pain. This suggests that pain is an isolated phenomenon that can be dialed down like our blood pressure. If we looked at back pain as having a pain generator that is identifiable and treatable in a minority of the cases and, in those more common cases, we focus on the brain's capacity to interpret the pain, we would be improve our results and save money.

This is the potential power of both empathetic paternalistic medicine and patient autonomy. Most physicians subscribe to partnering with their patients in decision-making. The idea that the physician is potentially capable of altering how the patient may actually feel may seem like a return to the dark ages. After all, medicine a century ago had little else to offer the patient. Was there not something positive there? Sure, we have discovered antibiotics and chemotherapy and technology has allowed us to image the body in great detail—all enhancing the capabilities of medicine—but with those changes, do we also abandon our power to sculpt our patients through contextualizing, rationalizing, and interpreting? Shakespeare famously said in *Hamlet*, "There's nothing either good or bad, but thinking makes it so."

Why not work both ends?

We—both the patient and the doctor—can with narrative medicine.

It is with that in mind, that we turn to learning the philosophy of narrative medicine.

PART III

THE PHILOSOPHY

Inside You'll Find:

Why Narrative Medicine Makes Sense in Science

The Biological Necessity of Narratives

The Sincerely Delusional Doctor

The Two Big Fat Greek Traits without Which We Cannot Practice Good Medicine

The Greek Traits of a Neurosurgeon

The Necessity of Transparency

The Formulation of Our Narratives

The power of a surgeon lies in his humanity and not his hands. This is not to discount the thousands of hours spent learning the technical aspects of the craft, but rather to highlight the equally demanding commitment to character development. Anyone with reasonable coordination could learn to perform neurosurgery with adequate competency. This acquired skill would suffice in the majority of situations. What allows a surgeon to standout, however, is his or her management of the patient. You have learned from the Promise section that this starts with the combined forces of empathetic paternalism and enhanced patient autonomy.

While the mere practice of medicine will allow for the development of character and an array of narratives, the point of this book is that mere practice is often not enough. Expression and transparency of what we have come to learn and believe is essential. This expression is particularly potent in the form of writing and teaching.

This section describes my personal journey. It weaves my experiences in medicine, and in life, with a lifelong fascination of philosophy. I left my undergraduate years wondering whether my interest in philosophy had any relevance. My perspective, thirty-five years later, is that philosophy represents the ideal antidote to the downside of technology. As medicine becomes more automated, computer-assisted, and commoditized, there is an increasing need for reflection, improvisation, inductive reasoning, and the challenging of the conventional wisdom. Embracing and incorporating philosophy promotes such endeavors and is the ideal foil for doctor overconfidence and money-driven practice habits.

Philosophers are natural reflectors, thinkers, and teachers. Before technology, they communicated and mused primarily through writing and public speaking, forming narratives that expressed the process that shape the character of mankind. Our narratives arise from the same processes that shape our character. While this is a natural process of living, like attaining a language, I believe that our narratives can be enhanced through the act of purposeful expression—reflection, writing, or teaching. This section of the book is meant to encourage a similar journey for you—one of a doctor becoming better doctor or a patient becoming better patient.

I include some philosophic principles that happen to be commonly derived from the Greek culture. This should not be surprising as the Greek philosopher, Hippocrates, is often considered the father of modern medicine. Hippocrates suggested that "wherever the art of medicine is loved, there is a love of Humanity." This is a peek into my humanity and my love of medicine.

CHAPTER 11

Narrative Medicine

To be human is to create narratives, but not all narratives are created equal. In health, it is the narrative that separates the good and great patient and the good and great doctor. In fact, I am going to try and convince you that the narrative is the essence of health.

Narrative medicine is the development of mental models on the part of doctors and patients. Mental models are developed not by the acquisition of facts, but quite the opposite. They are the mastering of general concepts. Facts, paradoxically, get in the way! Mental models require effort to develop. Doctors and patients need many different mental models to select from in order to be useful for a new problem. While this selection proves difficult, it provides a necessary flexibility and creativity.

Narrative medicine involves not only the development of these models, but the act of expression. For the doctor, this expression can be in the form of anecdotes, stories, and other teaching tools. For the patient, this expression is in the form of health habits and the formation of a comprehensive description of one's predicaments when they emerge.

For both doctors and patients, the narratives are empowered through a process of understanding biases. Biases undermine the development of narratives and the recognition of biases serves to empower the narratives. Similarly, the act of formal expression of our narratives can be empowering. This expression can be formal such as writing and teaching—preferable—or private through introspection or conversation.

It is the narrative that separates one doctor from another and one patient from another. Perhaps no other force has had a greater detrimental effect on our narrative than technology. While appearing to empower us (which it does), technology also undermines us by serving as a surrogate for face-to-face communication that allows the narrative of the doctor and the patient to intermingle and generate a new and empowered doctor-patient narrative.

Why Narrative Medicine Makes Sense in Science

"Words are, of course, the most powerful drug used by mankind."

—RUDYARD KIPLING, FROM A SPEECH HE MADE TO THE ROYAL COLLEGE OF SURGEONS IN LONDON, 1923

Nearly one hundred years ago, this author, journalist, and storyteller, most famous for his tale *The Jungle Book,* spoke to an audience of well-trained surgeons. Why invite a storyteller like Rudyard Kipling to offer advice and inspiration to a professional body of surgeons who had spent their lives performing medicine in ways no other humans on earth are equipped to do? Why not feature a highly regarded surgeon, the kind of icon that awards and scholarships are named for? It turns out a storyteller knows a hell of a lot more than we think about what makes good medicine. Storytelling relies on certain skills that are not focused on in medical school or in residency.

As I went through my seven-year apprenticeship as a neurosurgeon, I learned about the neurosurgical spectrum of diseases and the techniques used in the operating room to treat those diseases. I learned how to use a bayonetted forceps and how to coagulate tissue precisely between its tips. I figured out how to torque my thumb over the hole on a sucker to provide a graduated intensity of suction to the tissue.

But the first time I spoke with a family after a surgery, I was taken aback by the intensity of my audience. I had just spent seven years of my life honing my skills as a surgeon and the most recent three hours in using those skills operating, none of which the family was interested in hearing. Wanting to know exactly what just happened, I realized the family was in essence asking me to tell them a story, one in which the ending came first. However, depending on how good or bad that ending sounded, I would be required to fill in the beginning and middle. Herein lays the challenge; one that is evident in medicine day after day. Depending on the surgeon, the narrative approach can be construed and applied *very* differently. I could choose to embellish the story, so it goes in my favor (avoiding my wrongness). Even when the outlook was very good, and the surgery was an easy one, I could add some details that make it sound as if my job that day was harder than it actually was, martyring myself. Or, I could nuance the narrative to protect myself by telling the family what they wanted to hear rather than what actually happened—that perhaps pain post-op is something that is "normal," despite knowing it is a result of an unexpected slip up during the procedure. I could play the role of patriarch doctor, dictating to a family and patient what to do next with the insinuation that they are not interested in, nor capable of, being active participants in decision- making and care. I could save myself, and tell the family it was *their* call, and wash my hands of it all.

These are only a few options in a sea of possible narratives surgeons can choose from, but I didn't learn these languages overnight.

Naively, I had finished residency thinking that I had one weapon—a technical skill—and now, with this anxious family in the waiting room, I discovered that I had a second power: the ability to frame the operation or frame the way that I practice medicine, in any way I chose. How doctors frame the narrative was a large discussion of Part I: The Problem. I have learned that with great power comes great responsibility and so it hit me: the narrative was *my* story to tell. And it was my choice what kind of narrator I would be, even if nobody ever knew it but me—*especially* when nobody knew but me.

The argument of this book is that recognizing, adopting, and utilizing narrative medicine much as we do the technical, pharmacological, and surgical elements can make healthcare great again by mitigating the elements of The Problem outlined in this book and utilizing The Promises that are always right at our finger tips, if we choose to enforce them. But we need to be telling the right stories in the right contexts with the right intentions, becoming the kind of a narrators Kipling spoke of in his speech in 1923.

A good storyteller is an empathic person, who is filled with compassion, emotional intelligence, and maybe a little prescience. We already spoke a bit about empathetic paternalism, but one can only be truly engaged in this practice if the doctor, like storytellers, relies on being a mind reader, i.e., anticipating how the human psyche internalizes, contextualizes, and personalizes an occurrence. It is often about taking on, addressing, and accepting the perception of the others in lieu of your own perception of things.

In his quote, Kipling uses the metaphor of comparing words to drugs to illustrate how persuasive words can be to another person. As he says in the next line of his speech, "Not only do words infect, egotize, narcotize, and paralyze, but they enter into and color the minutest cells of the brain. . . ." What this means is that people have the ability to use words to change the way other people think and feel, to influence that person to do or feel things not typical for that person—just as drugs might do.

That is why the narrative is a part of medicine, as much a part as the technical and highly skilled part. As we have discussed in previous chapters, we can see how the medical establishment suffers when the narrative has gone missing. An essential role of the doctor is to convert facts into narratives through the promises of contextualization, biocentrism, heuristics, numeracy, and better decision- making. These narratives can be used in conversation with the patient in the form of stories, analogies, habits, etc. Effective storytelling is the key to influence. Effective influence is, in turn, an integral part of medical care—as important as selecting the ideal antibiotic.

Doctors are often lonely creatures. Although always around people, we are surprisingly alone. We carry on a silent and intensely personal dialogue that starts early in our training and follows along throughout our careers. The first step in creating our narratives is to tap into that dialogue. We are all vaguely aware of this voice in our heads, but when we sit down and bother to articulate it, its depth and intensity can be surprising. As we articulate it, it also begins to take shape and strengthen. As we articulate it, we, too, begin to take shape and strengthen.

The narrative is formed not so much from the facts we have originally learned, but from how we have uniquely come to practice. It is enhanced when we teach or mentor and, particularly, when we write. It is a personality of sorts, comprised of a balance between our instincts and the processes of our deep thinking, between what we have learned and original thought. It is a dynamic entity that is capable of growth. It must be both fair-minded and strong-minded. It must be memorable and resonate with our listeners.

Patients will frequently come into my office having suffered sudden and overwhelming back pain. Investigation into the etiology of their pain reveals little in the way of serious pathology and I attribute their pain to muscle spasm. In addition to explaining the teleological rational for muscle spasm, I share my own stories of experiencing similar intense pain. My personal experiences as a suffering patient provides the patient with many advantages when compared to an instructive explanation. It allows them to envision a positive ending. It provides empathy and understanding. It is an explanation buoyed with experience and containing a plan. The patients are motivated to listen to the story as it unfolds, eager to hear how it ends. They will remember the story much longer than the facts that I could have spewed out during the office visit. It is like remembering a person named Baker by associating them with the profession of baker. The name, Baker, is common and forgettable while the profession, baker, conjures up vivid images of pastries and, thus, stays with you.

Stories are told based on the perception of the narrator's reality—how he sees things based on conditioning, nature, nurture, and a host of other factors. Because of the different variables in an individual's life, we each tend to perceive reality much differently. "If things happen one way to you and the same things happen another way to me, then what is real? What stories, whose views, comprise reality?" While such a question goes beyond the scope of this book, weighing how differently a surgeon and a patient perceive the reality of their circumstances is critical to understanding the bridge between them and that bridge is precisely where the most effective paradigm of healthcare lies.

Additionally, the narratives or the internal stories, we tell ourselves about our circumstances, actions, and emotions, are far from being simple and straightforward. They are based on many biases and fallacies that can undermine our intentions. When our biases and fallacies are recognized and addressed, our narratives improve. Narrative medicine requires both doctors and patients to commit time to identifying how they decide and commit energy into improving their narratives.

The popular Showtime series *The Affair* illustrates that reality is in the eye of the beholder. The show depicts events as separately remembered by each participant (Noah and Allie). Not only do the motives and storyline differ, but even the basic "facts" such as how they were dressed are different. It poignantly reminds us that there is no reality, only perception. We touched briefly on the flaws and biases of decision-making in chapter 7. In medicine, one such common bias that distorts reality and interferes with our progress is confirmation bias—our need to align with facts that justify what we believe to be right and true or that lessen our guilt when we act out of line with our personal value system. This bias arises from our instinctual need to protect our beliefs. Interestingly, it is so powerful that when we are provided with information that contradicts what we believe, we not only ignore the new information, but we process it in such a way as to further solidify our original belief. This has been dubbed the backfire effect.

Patients routinely come into the office with beliefs that are derived from their particular upbringing or the overwhelming influence of our culture. I spend as much time disabusing patients of these notions as I do teaching the science of medicine.

It would be simplistic to view the doctor-patient encounter as sufficient if comprised only of communicating and applying the science of medicine. The narratives a doctor and a patient will tell themselves are as different as Noah and Allie's stories both of which are laced with bias. A more powerful way of viewing medicine acknowledges the patient and doctor as possessing separate perceptions of medicine, each distorted by a number of biases and fallacies. Even the science, itself, must be viewed as flawed—subject to change, or plain wrong, which is why I believe a healthy skepticism of science is part of The Promise. The doctor-patient relationship has the potential to transform these disparate perceptions into a more unified and useful perception by allowing narratives to flourish. Just as Allie and Noah carry distinctly different perceptions of events that they shared, neither one represents "reality." Just as there is an art to interpreting ancient texts, there is an art to interpreting medicine. There is no objective truth, only interpretations, and interpretations that are alive, dynamic, and subject to change. Combining two viewpoints, however, could potentially facilitate a more accurate reality than either could arrive at independently. In the story that you will read in chapter 17, I believe that is what I was able to achieve by assisting the family of the brain hemorrhage patient.

Mentalizing (mind reading) is at the core of the narrative. Separate parts of the brain light up when doing analytic thinking versus social thinking. Social thinking involves what is commonly looked at as the theory of the mind or the capacity to predict what someone else is thinking about something. This capacity to socialize is so important that we all possess a part of our brain that has been called the default network. With the creation of fMRIs (a technique to actually see which part of the brain is active during an activity), early experience noted that a part of our brain turned on after any purposeful activity had stopped. We now believe that this automatically occurring phenomenon is used to socially contextualize that which has just been experienced or learned.

In other words, we are hardwired to create narratives. Or, put another way, our need to share an experience is inexorably tied into that experience. To take it one step further, how we share the experience has the potential to enhance that experience. The creation of narratives in medicine thus can enhance the experience of medicine.

Creating a narrative makes us into information DJs. Just as a music DJ listens to music in a fundamentally different way than does the passive listener who listens only for enjoyment, formulating thoughts to be conveyed as narratives intensifies the narrator's experience and makes it transformative.

The narrative in medicine cannot simply be a regurgitation or distillation of what the literature suggests about a certain problem. It must utilize our abilities in mentation. We must use the part of our brain that projects how our patients will react to what we teach them and what we recommend. It must not only forecast what our patients are anticipating and would really like, but also when our patients misjudge how they think they will feel. There are many layers of this type of thinking. In chapter 12, we will discuss this as the Greek trait known as empathy.

The Sincerely Delusional Doctor

A colleague once articulated his recipe for spine surgery. "It's very simple," he said. "I identify the painful disc space, and then I fuse it." My immediate reaction to his simplistic and self-serving philosophy was frustration. He was clearly delusional, because identifying the painful disc (or whether it is even a disc that is causing the pain) is extremely difficult. In addition, even in cases where the pain generator seems quite evident, fusion fails to consistently yield good results. I knew that when it comes to a delusional person, there is no changing his mind. At the same time, I was impressed by his sincerity. There was no doubt that he earnestly believed in how he practiced medicine.

What do we make of a person who exhibits the great trait of sincerity along with the dangerous trait of delusion? At first glance, sincerity is appealing. It connotes honesty, but that is about all it does. In a scene in William Gaddis's novel *The Recognitions*, the immature playwright, Otto, defends his love for his friend Esme on a New York City street, saying, "You know I'm sincere … I've always been sincere."

Esme dismissively responds, "Sincerity becomes the honesty of people who cannot be honest with themselves."

This look inward is the essence of the narrative. It is not enough for the surgeon to be sincere; he must also be authentic and connected with his core values. It requires the doctor to transcend biases of his practice which he may be blind to or that he may have convinced himself are true, just as Noah remembers Allie being a seductress wearing all black while Allie remembers being dressed humbly and unknowingly pursued by Noah. My surgeon friend was guilty of the post hoc fallacy—the idea that because Y happened after X, X caused Y to happen. Since many of his patients *seemed* to be doing well after surgery, he could think that the surgery must be the proximate cause of their success. What he failed to consider was that many patients find a way to rationalize or muster optimism out of disappointing results. Do you remember the concept of biocentrism from the Promise section? Surprisingly, a patient doing well after an operation does not prove that the correct operation was done correctly. Part of how a patient is "doing" depends on many factors that include, but are not limited to, the removal of the painful stimulus. Pain, like so many of our basic sensations is not a simple representation of reality. Pain is processed and altered by our brains. While this may smell of ambiguity or pseudoscience, it also provides an opportunity for the surgeon. The surgeon may serve as a contextualizer, and as such, help influence the way the patient's brain processes and alters the pain.

More likely, with this delusional surgeon, his other patients who were not doing well and were not able to find a positive spin, either sought another doctor or were unwilling to let him know (remember Elmer, who gave me and my nurse two different answers to the question of his satisfaction?). Or, perhaps he was unable to listen to those who were not doing well (confirmation bias) in an act of hearing what supported what he wants to believe and not hearing that which was contradictory. Was this surgeon dishonest? He was flawed and guilty of bias, but not dishonest. He was sincere, but not authentic. He lacked two vital traits necessary for narratives and doing good medicine: humility (in this case the inability to embrace wrongness) and empathy.

CHAPTER 12

The Two Big Traits without Which We Cannot Practice Good Medicine

Case after case and year after year, I have worked with many surgeons who make the same mistakes as the Delusional Doctor I wrote about in the previous chapter. Their failure to change is often rooted in overconfidence. This is not surprising as these same surgeons use their overconfidence to build their practices. Patients are attracted to confident surgeons.

Early in my career, I noticed that if I presented what I considered an honest appraisal of the surgery by admitting that the results would be unpredictable (which was the truth), some patients would choose a different surgeon who had presented the same operation with more confidence, or shall I say, with more of a direct answer. My lesson became that patients would prefer to have the same surgery from a surgeon who "guaranteed" success. And so I learned to appear more reassuring and this was rewarded with more patients and more surgeries. One of the greatest parts of getting older (and there aren't that many) is that now I can return to the honest appraisal and not lose the patient. In fact, I have learned that the vast majority of patients actually do appreciate transparency and that includes admitting when I screw up and that I can never guarantee anything.

Humility (Embracing Wrongness)

I started to think of wrongness and its relationship to medicine while reading *Being Wrong*: *Adventures in the Margin of Error* by Kathryn Schulz. In her wonderful, philosophical treatise, she underscores the benefits of embracing wrongness. Why not apply this to medicine as well? After all, medicine is a field obsessed with not being wrong.

When on call as a medical student I was awakened by my resident and asked to perform a finger stick on well-to-do patient. Typically, a more senior member of the team would have performed this task, but they were all busy. It was early in my career and I had not yet mastered the technique of performing without completely waking up. This particular time, to maintain orientation in my sleeping state, I repeated the task to myself—a kind of mantra—while I made my way to the patient. Unbeknownst to me, the words became jumbled in my sleep and "finger stick" was transformed to "stick finger."

Several minutes later, rather than pricking the patient's finger to get a reading of her blood glucose level (finger stick), I did a rectal exam and checked the patient for blood in the stool. I dutifully documented my actions and slipped back to sleep.

The next morning, the ritual of rounds progressed in the traditional way. There was an attending, several residents, and the lowly medical student, yours truly. Since this patient had some sort of status, which I didn't understand, the attending physician spent a good deal of time speaking with her. At the end of the visit he asked her if she had any questions. You bet she did. "Just one," she said, looking over at me. "Why did that young man— and everyone turned to look at me as she was pointing—wake me up in the middle of the night to do a rectal exam?" Yes, to err is human, and yet, this is not acceptable in medicine. In the mind of the doctor, to err is shameful and punishable, and in this moment I felt no different. As a consequence, there is no embracing of being wrong. There is an avoidance of being wrong. There is an effort to cover up when wrong or to avoid situations in which being wrong is more probable. These tendencies seem to protect the individual doctor in the short run, but undermine his development over time.

Schulz points out that being wrong has a real upside. If you watch children learn, you will see that they do a lot of trial and error. They seem to look at error as a source of growth and not a failure. How often do we say that you can't learn to ski without falling down, but do we really allow ourselves to fall down in medicine? Not with the current medical-legal climate. There is a legal system in place that rewards patients for doctor's errors. It does this by vilifying the doctors that are involved in these errors. I understand that there has to be a system of monitoring the practice of doctors. This creates accountability and is protective of the patient, but if the patient's protection is the true bottom line, then the system backfires. The current system is clearly too much of a business. It is not patients who benefit, but lawyers. Patients are punished by the constraining forces put on the doctors. Too many tests are ordered. Communication goes from being educational to protective. The current system is not good enough at distinguishing between what is human error and what is negligence.

Politicians have mitigated this distinction through the use of clever semantics. One rarely hears, "I was wrong," but more often, "Mistakes were made." If that was the way in which mistakes in medicine were conceived, we would be more willing and able to embrace our mistakes and, in turn, learn from them. This would not preclude financial remuneration for those patients that deserve such, or punitive measures for truly negligent doctors.

Medical legal issues aside, I would like to advocate for the embracing of wrongness by the physician as a personal philosophical mandate. Overconfidence in the surgeon can be a fatal flaw. Schulz points out that certainty is the enemy of creativity and empathy. I would add that certainty is also the enemy of personal growth. The best convictions are not without doubt but in spite of doubt.

Babies add the word "maybe" to their repertoire of answers at age five, which includes only "yes" and "no" before that time. This is presumably a cognitive milestone that acknowledges that life is not only lived in the spirit of black and white, but with many shades of gray. Similarly, the doctor also needs to add to his repertoire the answer "maybe," or, better yet, "I don't know but I can find out," or even the impossible, "I was wrong."

Patients should also take heed. Part of what drives the doctor to offer a black-and-white answer is pressure from the patient, which we discussed a bit in The Problem. Patients are not comfortable with ambivalence—even when it is appropriate. Part of embracing wrongness is to accept an *aporetic* nature of reality. This is a Greek term that refers to arguments that have more than one right answer. For example, most situations in medicine have more than one good treatment.

As doctors, we have a tendency to listen to the patient just long enough to formulate our response. Once we formulate it in our mind, we can barely wait for the patient to end speaking so we can jump in. We stop listening when our own mental formulation occurs. This ultimately limits the power of the exchange. Accepting wrongness allows us to listen to the patient's full story and that is how the narrative develops.

Complications and Mistakes

I found myself alone in the operating room taking out a tumor from the frontal lobe of a young woman's brain. The patient had presented to the emergency room with a seizure. She had no insurance and no family. She was profoundly schizophrenic, so not much history could be attained.

The attending surgeon assigned to the case thought it would be a good teaching case. He, as well as the radiologists, presumed it was a malignant tumor. It was a massive tumor growing into both frontal lobes from just above the orbit (the bony encasing for the eye).

I was at work removing the frontal sinus, which is an aerated part of the bone that would need to be removed to get adequate exposure for the tumor removal. As I took out the contents of the frontal sinus, I remember feeling a sense of satisfaction. I was entrusted to take care of this patient and I had been trained to take care of the frontal sinus a couple of times in the past. This great feeling, however, was replaced with a sense that something may be wrong. I had taken out the contents of the frontal sinus before, but was this material I was removing different? I slowed up and reoriented myself. I asked the question that comes up a lot in surgery, "Am I doing the right thing?"

Suddenly the good feelings were abruptly replaced with visceral panic and nausea. I realized that I may have been in the orbit and what I thought was sinus contents may have been the eyeball! I called for the attending who scrubbed in and surveyed the situation. "You are fine," he told me, but he had not looked carefully enough and I was not convinced.

Ultimately, it became clear that I had been in the orbit. I didn't take out the eyeball, but the patient ended up blind in that eye after surgery. What was presumed to be a malignant tumor ended up being a benign tumor. This tumor would not end her life, making her blindness a lifelong affliction.

For the first time I had experienced a sinking feeling that unfortunately is familiar to all surgeons on occasion. It is an intense sense of dread when one becomes aware that he has just done something terrible to a patient and that the harm done was a mistake. Mistakes are different than complications. Complications are recognized possible bad outcomes related to the procedure, while mistakes suggest bad outcomes related to surgeon errors.

This occasional feeling is one of the hardest things about being a surgeon. It lasts for days, or sometimes, weeks. It comes down like a sledgehammer and blunts any type of happiness. Complications are part of neurosurgery. As such, we are destined to experience the powerful emotional effects throughout our careers.

Mistakes are more difficult to swallow than complications. Sometimes we make mistakes that don't result in patient harm. This is due to either luck, or more commonly, to the remarkable ability of the human body to heal and adapt. Since unrecognized mistakes are not punishable, they are more easily swept under the carpet. If complications and mistakes were both used for the purposes of self-improvement, we would grow more efficiently. Humility is the means by which we acknowledge not only our complications and mistakes, but those mistakes that are inconsequential to the patient.

In this case, there was no complication reported or acknowledged because the patient had no family and impaired cognition. There was a mistake made, however, and one that I will never make again (hopefully) and one that I learned from. When mistakes occur, they loom over us for days. I try to rationalize them by remembering that I was trying my hardest, but it doesn't really work. I often am overwhelmed by the feeling that I shouldn't even be a neurosurgeon. The mistakes hauntingly enter surgeons' consciousness over and over again. Sometimes my mind plays out the scene like a song stuck in my mind. I am also trapped in a mood, so that nothing seems enjoyable. It is similar to the death of a loved one, with our thoughts returning to the issue as a default location. It may leave our consciousness for a brief period of time, but the essence and mood looms over us like a pall.

I have been in the dumps many times in over my nearly thirty years as a surgeon. It is the single worst part of being a surgeon. You may think that our triumphs neutralize our complications, but that is not the case. It is a condition that is ours to bear and it doesn't get easier over time. No wonder our instinct is to avoid this feeling, but trying to avoid it is not only impossible but counterproductive. At some point, we all have to look at our skill as a work in progress. Complacency is disingenuous and cockiness is shortsighted, as looking back will always shine a diminutive light on what we do now. This is part of how we grow. It is partly from our mistakes that our narratives take root.

Would I trade my guilty conscience for peace of mind? Never. I remind myself that my humanity, my errors, my embracing wrongness are what keep me fully human, and it is in being human that I can tap my biological need to connect with other humans through the character trait known as empathy. Without my humility, I could not engage in empathetic paternalism, and without that, the ability to form narratives is impossible.

Empathy

As a third-year resident I took off on a Saturday morning for a several hour day trip to visit an institutionalized patient with severe hydrocephalus and to answer a most interesting consultative question. I had been asked whether I could make a young man's skull smaller. It turns out that the child was born with hydrocephalus. This particular condition resulted in the child producing more spinal fluid than he could reabsorb. If this occurs as an adult, the pressure in the skull will increase. If it occurs in a child before the skull has formed, the skull will continue to grow and grow.

This child had been abandoned by his parents and institutionalized. He was presumed to be severely retarded and nothing was done for his hydrocephalus. His head had become enormous. So enormous that he was unable to lift it off of the bed. It weighed around ninety pounds and the patient would just pivot around bed with his head stuck on the mattress due to its weight (a typical head is eighteen pounds).

I knew before going to see him that I would not be able to help, but something in me wanted to witness the situation in person.

My motivation, which had been a morbid curiosity, was abruptly altered when I stood in the presence of this child. Aside from feeling pathetic from letting my curiosity trump my compassion, I was filled with an overwhelming sense of empathy.

There is no way that reading about this child or even seeing pictures of this child would have been able to invoke such a strong sensation. For days I couldn't stop thinking about the child. Twenty-five years later I still hold the memory and the intensity of my reaction.

We, as humans, are hard-wired for empathy. Modern science is unraveling the biologic basis of empathy from studies in psychology and from fMRI. A picture of our brain as a social structure has emerged. We have known for some time from the use of PET scans that after finishing a cognitive, motor, or visual task, our brains turn on a region which has been called the default network. This is consistently activated when we are "doing nothing." It turns out that our brains are far from doing nothing. This default network is a process of taking our recent activity, contextualizing it socially, and making sense of how the new information fits into our self-perception and our perceptions of others. It is likely something that we are hardwired to do. It has likely developed because of its survival advantage. Not all of our survival advantages have to do with competition for survival; some are related to cooperation and the social brain can play an invaluable part in such behavior.

Humans may not be the strongest or fastest of animals, but our capacity to socialize allows us to better protect ourselves against the forces of nature. Perhaps our social capacity develops similarly to our visual system. Without effort, we transform light and color into progressively complicated images, not by trying, but simply by living. One of the theories of why our brains are proportionally large relative to our body size when compared with other mammals is in our capacity to develop social relationships. This is further supported by the fact that much of our brain growth takes place after we have left the womb, allowing our social interactions to influence the development.

Our shared thoughts and social nature are not only a survival advantage, but a source of pleasure and pain that is uniquely human. This pleasure has been tied to something called essentialism. This is the pleasure that is derived simply from the knowledge that a real person is involved. For example, we will pay money for a shirt actually worn by a celebrity. Even though that shirt is, in itself, indistinguishable from any other similar shirt, the fact that it was worn by someone increases its value and the pleasure that can be derived from it. If you were to purchase a Picasso for more than a million dollars and spent five minutes staring at it each time you left the house—to attain pleasure—how would you feel if you discovered it was a counterfeit? Even though the picture would look the same, the pleasure from looking at it would vanish. This is essentialism. The difference between immense pleasure and minimal pleasure is simply controlled by our knowledge of who painted the picture. This is a powerful manifestation of our social brains. It is the force that allows us to look at other people, not as generic parts of a crowd, but as unique and remarkable individuals filled with essentialism.

Similarly, with this enhanced connectedness, there is enhanced vulnerability. We are susceptible to heartbreak. Almost every doctor can tell a story of medical heartbreak. Mine occurred with an aneurysm patient. I was the junior resident and responsible for admitting her to the floor after she suffered a small bleed into the fluid space around her brain. After explaining to her that she would need surgery because the bleed suggested that she was at a heightened risk for another bleed, she asked, "Why wait until tomorrow?" I explained to her the balance between wanting to get it done as quickly as possible and wanting a well-rested surgeon and experienced operating room team. She asked me to promise her that she would be okay overnight, which I did.

You can probably guess that she died suddenly overnight from a re-hemorrhage. I was heartbroken. I vowed to never allow myself to get attached to a patient. I justified this plan by convincing myself that I would be a better clinician were I to remove the emotions from my decision-making. Part of my personal growth as you will learn is in recognizing how wrong this is. Empathy is essential and although it carries the risk of pain, the other rewards far outweigh that drawback. It is better to have loved and lost than to have never loved.

In *Social: Why Our Brains Are Wired to Connect* by Matthew D. Lieberman, empathy is depicted as requiring three components. First, is our capacity to mentalize. This is our ability to guess what is in the mind of another. Much has been written about mirror neurons. This is the part of our brain that fires when we watch another perform an activity. It even fires when we think of performing that same activity. Lieberman thinks that while our vision tells us what is going on, the mirror neurons help us to understand how it is happening. Mentalizing is one step further. It helps to tell us why it is happening.

In addition to mentalizing, we need to affect share. This is our capacity to imagine what another is feeling. This is closest to what many imagine that empathy is—a shared feeling. Finally, there is one last step—taking action. What allows us to not only see the why, feel the pain, but to then take action? Most of the time we find ourselves busy and able to suppress the empathetic feelings we have. Lieberman suggests that the septal part of our brain is responsible for prompting action. This is the part of a mother's brain that allows her to tend to her distressed child.

Given our hard-wired, natural gifts of empathy, you can

understand why I often say that I have the easiest job in the world. All I have to do is use my body of knowledge and my years of experience to predict what is best for the patient. But how do I actually get inside of my patient's head? Being a good doctor requires empathy. Is this something one either has or doesn't have or can it be developed?

If I can understand what my patients want or believe, do I prioritize their desires? What if I really think that what they want is a mistake? Henry Ford was quoted as saying, "If I asked my customers what they wanted, they would have told me a faster horse." This represents yet another tension in medicine—balancing what the patient wants or thinks is right with what the doctors believes is best.

When we were young we were taught the Golden Rule: "Do onto others as they would do onto you." Empathy asks us to modify this rule to what has been called the Platinum Rule: "Do onto others what they would have you do onto them." The latter doesn't fully apply to medicine, as the doctor has something of value that the patient doesn't always understand. Empathetic paternalism is the process by which the doctor nudges the patient beyond the Platinum Rule- "Do onto others what you have shown them that they would have you do onto them."

Empathy can also be altered in medicine by the doctor's sense of medical-legal vulnerability.

I was covering one of my pediatric colleagues when I was called to see a five-year-old boy with a ventriculoperitoneal shunt (a tube that connects the fluid cavities of the brain with the cavity that contains the bowels) who was lethargic. When children have such a shunt placed they are often, thereafter, in a precarious position. They can become dependent on the shunt and thus vulnerable if the shunt malfunctions. This vulnerability can even be life-threatening. When the pediatrician called me to say that the boy didn't look right, I took his assessment very seriously. I examined the boy who did appear to be lethargic. I went out to the waiting area to speak with his mother. She was a single mother who was clearly devoted to her son. I explained to her that we would do a CT scan to assess her son's ventricular size and shunt function.

She was the kind of mother that I immediately liked and formed a bond with. Sometimes in medicine you simply connect with patients and their families. You can come emotionally invested in a short period of time. While I was speaking with her, I was paged back to the ICU. The boy had become unresponsive. A quick examination revealed a serious deterioration in the level of consciousness. When I examined the boy, he appeared to be brain dead.

I have seldom seen such an abrupt deterioration. He went from lethargic to brain dead in just a few minutes. While I was deciding what to do, I looked up and saw his mother. She was staring in disbelief and in agony. I decided to place a drain into the ventricles without even getting a CT scan. I was able to place the drain, but the pressure was only mildly elevated. A follow up CT was not helpful. I felt helpless as I watched the boy die. The mother was there next to me unable to say anything.

For weeks after the event I was haunted. Had I missed something? Could I have done something different? I also felt as if the mother was disappointed in me. I am not a pediatric neurosurgeon and I wondered if she thought that having a pediatric neurosurgeon would have resulted in a different outcome. I wanted to write her a note saying how sorry I was, but part of me resisted this urge as I worried that it may be perceived as a token of guilt.

It reminded me of this peculiar anxiety I had while in college. I would be walking toward a door to enter a building and, at the same time, be aware that there was a female student behind me. It always seemed that the distance was just enough to make it awkward. If I went through the door and didn't hold it, I was being rude. If I walked through the door and held it, I was being solicitous. I remember slowing down or speeding up to avoid this dilemma. Looking back, I wish I had the confidence to open the door, look behind me while holding it, and say "take your time."

Similarly, I wished I had written the patient's mother a quick note. I shouldn't have worried about what reaction she would have, but should only have focused on what I wanted to share. Three months after the incident, the mother wrote me a note. She thanked me for my efforts and let me know that she understood that everything that could have been done was done. I vowed that I would never again hold back a gesture that I believed in. Each of these incidents remind me that, in life, we are much more likely to regret what we have not done than what we have done.

What stopped me from fully exercising my empathy was a lack of self-confidence that stemmed from medical-legal vulnerability. Part of maturing as a surgeon is being willing to say what is on your mind as opposed to what you think the patient would want to hear.

Empathy is also dampened by the surgeons' pride. So much of our training emphasizes the critical role we play as we use our hands to take on the patient's health issue. Some of our training should be in learning to say "I don't know" or considering that we are not going to be the best at everything and that's OK.

Early in my career, I had two aneurysms in two different patients to clip in one day. The first was the patient of one of my senior partners. I was to be the assistant in this case. We had never done an aneurysm together and I was curious as to how my partner stacked up against the mentors who had trained me.

As the case progressed, I watched my partner in awe. He did a more thorough dissection than I had been taught to do in residency. When he had finished the dissection of the aneurysm, he moved the fragile dome back and forth to show me all sides and aspects of the aneurysm. He then, anticlimactically, placed a clip across the neck and we were done.

The next case was my patient and my senior partner would be the assistant. Rather than do the case as I had been trained, I set out to do the same dissection as my partner has done. I had finished this and then began to eagerly show him all parts of the aneurysm.

In my effort to duplicate what he had done, the aneurysm ruptured. This is not typically an issue when the neck and anatomy have already been worked out, but this rupture was at the neck of the aneurysm and required a different clip. This clip would need to encircle the parent vessel in order to secure the aneurysm. This encircling clip ended up compromising the parent vessel slightly.

When the patient awoke, I discovered that she had some mild weakness of her leg. Follow-up imaging revealed a small stroke, undoubtedly related to my technical flaw.

The patient was an older Italian woman who was part of a large, warm family. She and the extended family had been beside themselves with fear prior to the surgery. Their fears involved mainly her dying during the procedure. When the patient became aware of her postoperative deficit, she was barely perturbed. After all, she was alive.

I learned very quickly that day that making a mistake is far less forgivable when that mistake is made out of inexperience or naiveté. My mistake, however, was the result of being cavalier and in an attempt to impress. Forgiving oneself proves to be much more difficult in this setting.

Of course, to make things worse, the patient loved me. She would walk into the office beaming and telling her family, "This is the doctor who saved my life." All I could think was, *No, this is the doctor who gave you a stroke while trying to impress my partner.*

Part of me wanted to confess and disabuse her of her thankfulness. Part of me wanted to be punished. In general, I am an advocate of transparency and telling the truth, but what if the truth is not what is best for the patient. What if my confession served no positive purpose and only served to undermine the positive feelings and positive spin that the patient had constructed in her analysis of the surgery. Besides, her praise was punishment enough.

Empathy can also be contaminated by technology. Facebook or other social media sites would seem to have the potential to magnify our empathy by exposing us to more and different lives, but the medium serves to blunt the poignancy.

One of the interesting ways in which Facebook influences our social relationships is by forcing us to have a consistent persona. Rather than being a certain way with one friend and another way with a different friend, by posting publicly, we are forced into a single persona. Part of the nuance and power of empathy is to adapt our persona in each different environment. By collapsing our personas into one persona, we lose some of our empathy resilience.

In addition, the aspects of socialization that require touch, taste or smell are missing. There is an empathy hierarchy. Words are good, stories are better, pictures and sounds better yet, but one-on-one, in-person encounters are the best.

CHAPTER 13

The Greek Traits of a Neurosurgeon

I have an image etched into my brain from a night I was being held captive (on call) in the middle of my residency. It was a Saturday night and I was scheduled for the entire weekend. There was a big party that night that all of my friends would be attending and I was feeling a little sorry for myself.

I was coming to the end of my "junior years" a period during which I had been on call nearly every other night. This particular night had been difficult. It was 3:00 in the morning and I had no prospect for sleep. As the night went on, my "to do" list became progressively longer despite my hurried attempt to keep up with the flow from the emergency room.

As I walked alone down the hallway of the hospital, I was overcome with emotion. "This sucks!" I felt like screaming. I was tired, overwhelmed, and burned out. Consumed with self-pity, I had a moment of clarity. I thought to myself, "Take a mental picture of tonight, one that includes the fatigue, the pain, and the pressure. Emblazon it so that becomes indelible in your mind. If later in life you find yourself successful, don't feel guilty. Remember that this is what you had to go through."

Amazingly, I have revisited that scene many times over the years. Although the raw feeling has softened over time, the emblazoned memory serves as a mantra of sorts, which I visit when I feel guilty about my current success.

The process of becoming a neurosurgeon doesn't end, but it does get easier. Neurosurgeons share certain traits that we either acquire through the intensity of our residency or perhaps we always possessed them and they were the impetus that collectively guided us into neurosurgery. The stereotypical neurosurgeon is confident, perhaps even arrogant. He can cope with life and death issues with a necessary detachment. He is a unique blend of technophile and artisan. But there are some other traits that you may not associate with neurosurgeons. I have found some of these traits captured in the words of the ancient Greeks.

Praxis

Praxis refers to the action part of a process. Aristotle used the word *praxis* to distinguish it from the theoretical part of the process. In neurosurgery, patients with a condition called normal pressure hydrocephalus exhibit the opposite of praxis, or what we call, apraxia, inertia. When watching these patients walk, it looks like their feet are magnetically pulled into the floor. They have the strength to walk, the will and knowledge to walk, but they have difficulty walking, nonetheless. Their feet drag along the floor. Praxis suggests just the opposite—the ability to act, even when knowing what to do or how to do it is missing.

Early in my career, I was involved in the removal of a difficult meningioma. Although this is typically a benign tumor, it can be intimately attached to the brain so that its removal can injure the brain surface to which it is attached. This tumor was located between the two hemispheres of the brain and near the part of the brain responsible for controlling the movement on the opposite side of this patient's body. The tumor was large and deep so that it was not visible on the surface of the brain once the necessary portion of skull was removed and the covering of the brain was opened. This tumor had parasitized the vascularity that would typically supply the brain. Its removal required microsurgical technique to assure that the tumor was separated not only from the brain but also in a way that allowed preservation of the blood supply to the brain.

This patient had presented with a seizure during her pregnancy and had been scheduled to undergo the surgery shortly after she had given birth. She and her husband were understandably nervous about the operation as they were in that wonderful part of life where they were newly married, starting careers, and blessed with their first baby.

While I was removing the tumor I had the microscope zoomed all of the way up to better see the small blood vessels and allow me to stay in the plane between the tumor and the vessels of the brain. Sometimes a microscope zoomed to such a high power sacrifices the larger picture in order to provide such detail. In this case I lost the forest while focusing on the trees. I zoomed out the microscope only to realize that the brain had mushroomed out of the skull by more than 3 inches.

This was the result of edema, excess water content in the brain, and swelling that the tumor had produced. This is not an unusual finding, but I had never experienced this degree of swelling. It was obvious that I would not be able to place the bone back over the brain at the end of the case. Fortunately, I had learned several "tricks" to mitigate this situation such as hyperventilating the patient, giving a sugar called mannitol into the patient's blood, and raising the head of the bed.

This time, these efforts made no impact on the swelling.

I was filled with that sudden sense of dread that every neurosurgeon is well aware of. The sudden realization that, this person, who had put her faith in me, was in big trouble—and I was responsible. There was no way to close either the bone or the scalp over this mushroomed brain. The patient was going to die, or at very least, be impaired. I was going to have to amputate some of her brain to close the wound.

I wanted one of my mentors to come in and tell me what to do. Do I sacrifice brain to close? What do I tell her husband who is nervously pacing in the waiting room? This is a "benign" tumor. What will the staff in the room think of me if I harm a young and healthy woman with a benign tumor?

I had used up my bag of tricks and my mind was suddenly numb. I began to rehearse my pending conversation with the patient's husband. "I'm sorry. We lost her on the table." That is the strange thing about surgery. We learn early that an integral part of every case takes place after the case is finished. It is the conversation with the family. As my mind returned to the task at hand, I thought of one last thing that I could try. I called my partner to see if he could crawl underneath the drapes and sterilely place a needle into the patient's spinal canal in order to drain the spinal fluid from around the brain in which the brain floats. Fortunately, as spinal fluid flowed through the needle into a sterile bag, the brain began to settle into the cranium. I was greatly relieved.

Now, I had another decision to make. Should I quit while ahead and simply close or should I continue with the operation and take out the rest of the tumor. If I went for more tumor resection, the same swelling could occur again. Again, my mind went to the waiting area where her husband waited. I pictured the disappointment on his face when I told him that I couldn't remove the entire tumor. I decided to finish the case.

Fortunately, the patient awakened intact and had a relatively uneventful postoperative course.

When the patient was more than a month out from surgery and out of danger, I decided to tell her and her husband what had happened. My motive was to let them know how lucky we all were. Sometimes, a brush with death can allow us to not sweat the small stuff and enjoy life more. Eventually, that is how they would come view the events of the surgery, but at the time I told them the story of the surgery all her husband could say, over and over, was, "holy shit."

At that moment when a surgeon realizes that there is no one to come to the rescue, he must take responsibility. Over the years, this has become almost second nature. I realize that if I were to fail at that endeavor I would be violating the trust that the patient put in me prior to the surgery. We don't have the right to avoid our responsibility. We have to choose a course of action—we must invoke *praxis*.

Thymos

Plato liked to divide our motivation into reason, eros (erotic love) and thymos (which is our self-esteem, purpose, or inner need for recognition).

Thymos is what truly motivates the neurosurgeon. *Thymos* was originally used to describe that which motivated a soldier to per-form a heroic act of sacrifice during a battle. This may suggest an excess of grandeur but seems to best encapsulate what motivates me to spend the necessary time with my patients or return to the hospital to speak with a family in despair.

Spending hours being a neurosurgeon doesn't make sense. We know that we should be home with our families or enjoying the parts of life that our privileged salary would permit and yet we often find ourselves overwhelmed, exhausted, and engaged in our business. This thymotic motivation is at the core of the neurosurgeon.

Years ago, when on call for the weekend, I had scheduled an elective simple herniated disc case. This particular day was busy and I asked the operating room to allow my patient to go into the room. I was finishing up in the ER and I felt that I would have enough time to see her prior to having general anesthesia.

An unexpected issue arose in the ER and I was called by the operating room to let me know that the patient was asleep and they were waiting for me. Mildly miffed at myself for not at least saying hello, I hurried to start my case.

When I arrived, I helped to turn the patient onto the prone position and began to focus on the task at hand. I put the MRI up on the view box and instantly saw the herniated disc. It was at the bottom-most disc space and on the left side. I checked with the nurses and the preoperative consent form and was startled when they both assured me that the pain was on the right side. I looked over my notes and verified that the pain was right-sided and the nurse was emphatic that she had asked the patient about her pain and it was all in the right leg.

The patient was now asleep and I had to make a decision. I could awaken the patient and ask her again, but she had just been asked and even in my preoperative consult, I had written that she had stated that she had right-sided pain.

What really bothered me was that I would have normally made a big deal about pain being on one side and the disc on the other side when I had originally seen her. On occasion, a disc may be eccentric to the opposite side, and, on occasion, I have operated on such patients when I believed that there was no other explanation for their pain. More often than not, these patients fared well. In this case there was no such documentation and no suggestion that I had looked at this case other than as a straight-forward disc herniation. Something was wrong.

I cursed myself for being careless. I understood that my volume had reached a dangerous level and that I would have to make changes, but this would be dealt with later. I had to make a decision now (praxis).

Ultimately, I decided to approach the side of the pain and not what the MRI told me. As I exposed the nerve root I was praying that I would find something more than the MRI suggested. As soon as I began to mobilize the nerve root I knew that there was a disc herniation and that the patient was going to feel better. The herniation was, in fact large and impressive. I removed it and felt a huge sense of relief.

After the case, I was dictating what I had done and what I had found as I simultaneously looked at the MRI. I suddenly realized that the MRI showed that the disc was indeed on the right. I simply had gotten confused between left and right.

MRIs have always had an unusual orientation. Left is right and right is left, but this was something that I had dealt with many times in the past.

Why did I get confused that day?

I was under a lot of pressure to cover the emergency room as well as to finish my elective operating schedule for the week. I had only had a few hours of sleep the night before. But these, too, were conditions that I frequently experienced.

To someone who has never done surgery it may seem unimaginable that such a basic mistake could be made, but for a surgeon such a mistake is very easy to make. Abstract ideas such as left or right provide little content to the meaning of a case. In this case the OR checklist ultimately saved me from a devastating mistake.

I was saved by the nurses who I had long since learned to trust. We have "time outs" in the operating room, but the surgeon's mind is not always open to change and the time out may not free him from that conviction. Escaping in this case was the result of my own humility and the system of teamwork put in place.

Thymos is the force that makes us work, work, work. Humility allowed me the opportunity to reflect, reset my objectives, and create a new narrative. I would slow down and become more patient-centric

Apatheia

As a surgeon, I am often forced to enter a state of *apatheia*. This word derives its meaning similarly to apathy. But the meaning is quite different.

Picture this scene from my residency:

I am in the zone, as we say in sports. I am working my way through a fissure (natural fold) in the brain, dissecting the arteries under a microscope on my way to a brain aneurysm. The patient on the table presented the day before with a ruptured aneurysm so that I am all too aware of the fragility of its dome and how careful my dissection must be.

I hear no sounds and I am not aware of time passing—I just focus. I have to bear in mind two things: 1) the aneurysm may cataclysmically rupture at any moment and 2) if it does, I have a very limited time to identify the pertinent anatomy while I control the rapid bleeding of the rupture. This is the most time-pressured and intense experiences that neurosurgeons must endure.

I have learned to adapt in this moment with *apatheia*. Although this word shares Greek roots with the work apathy, it could not be more different in connotation. Apathy suggests a lack of emotion. My emotions are flying. Apathy connotes a sense of detachment. I couldn't be more engaged. *Apatheia* is better described as a voluntarily imposed composure, one that allows both equanimity and focus. It maximizes our capacity for *praxis*. If the aneurysm bursts, panic will result in a poor outcome for the patient. *Apathiea* is a place that I must visit during the critical times in an operation.

As a surgeon involved in the critical part of a surgical case, *apatheia* serves both as an invaluable refuge and as a medium to bring about insight. It is useful when dealing with an emergency. When I do not get sucked up into the surrounding emotional turmoil, I can be more effective. I suppose that I may appear cold and clinical while operating in this space, but I know that it is a necessary place to inhabit on occasion. The team around me will respond with a similar calm and focus.

Apathiea is not a natural place to be. Again, its implementation is a narrative. In this case, it is nothing written, but a habit arrived at through reflection and practice.

Pronoia

Pronoia is a term dubbed by psychologists to describe a state of mind that is opposite to paranoia—that those around us are plotting to benefit us. To me it is a necessary state of mind to survive as a neurosurgeon.

Our discipline is filled with patients in pain, patients in fear, and patients with terminal conditions. Our organ of focus, the nervous system, is unique among organs and although orthopedic surgeons may jokingly say that the heart exists to pump blood to the bones, it is not a stretch to suggest that the heart's purpose is to support the brain. It is the essence of what we are. If we were to transplant our brain to another patient, that patient would not be the recipient of our brain. We would be the recipient of that patient's body.

Given the high stakes, it is essential that we adopt a lofty and Panglossian outlook of the world—one that is optimistic in the face of hardship. Our focus cannot be on what others are doing or what they may think, but only on what we are doing.

Sometimes I sit in the office and sense that none of my patients are doing well. I recognize this as a bias. Those that have gotten better are enjoying life while those that are still searching for improvement will come back. I have to believe that there are many of my patients thriving in the community or I would be overwhelmed by a sense of futility.

I can effectively do an operation for pain and find that my patient is not feeling better. My reasoning was sound, my operation went well, but the patient is not satisfied. It is difficult to not beat myself up in these situations. I must learn to be satisfied with doing my best. I must believe that my patients understand that I did my best and that neurosurgery is not perfect.

I have learned to approach my responsibilities with *pronoia*. Again, this is not natural. It is part of a narrative created to make me a better doctor. In Adam Grant's book *Give and Take: Why Helping Others Drives Our Success*, the world conceptually is divided into three types of people: givers, takers, and matchers. He points out that across industries and professions, givers often find themselves at the bottom of their respective fields. These givers appear to "turn the other cheek" so that they can be slapped again.

Who then, he asks, ends up on top? Takers or matchers? It turns out that the answer is neither. It is, again, givers. This revelation didn't surprise me. How does this apply to me as a surgeon? I have always been paid well for my services—often too well! How do I function as a giver then? Of course, I do charity work and take care of the indigent, but this is an obligation that comes with my profession and not a true lifestyle.

The answer is simple, actually. As any healthcare provider ponders treatment options for the patient, he must ultimately recommend what he views as the best treatment. But what is best? Most of the choices of treatment that we select from do not have a proven superiority. In this ambiguous setting, it is easy to fall into a self-serving routine. This is best exemplified in the 1966 quote from Abraham Maslow, "When all you have is a hammer, everything looks like a nail."

If you ask your barber if you need a haircut, he will answer "yes." This is an earnest answer in that it reflects the way he sees the world. He is being sincere, but not authentic.

The essence of being a "giver," in contrast, is to extract a rec-ommendation from the ambiguity that arises from the perspective of the patient and not the provider. Put more plainly, being a giver is to consider and address the reality/perception of the patient *before* the doctor placates his or her own reality, with knowledge that medicine is like living inside multiple world theory, where one universe inhabited by a doctor, and the other a patient, have converged.

Just as Grant suggests, giving is a recipe for success. Medicine is ultimately a word-of-mouth referral occupation. Giving, by tak-ing into account the perspective and needs of the patient, is met with appreciation, trust, and referrals. The recipe for creating the doctor-patient narratives is similar. If what the doctor gives the patient is what is best for the patient and the patient has bothered to learn about his problem and considered his many options, the patient will benefit and the doctor will ultimately get more refer-rals. If I am rendered transparent and focus on giving, I believe that my patients, coworkers, and students will conspire to make me happy.

CHAPTER 14

Transparency and a Rising Tide

When I operate, the image of my working hands is crisply displayed on a screen for the nurses, students, and anesthesiologists to view. Positioning of the patients, potential difficulties of the case, and special needs are similarly stated aloud so that the entire OR team is involved, a dialogue encouraged to stay opened. In turn, the nurses feel comfortable challenging anything that is being done or proposed. One might think this is a disastrous case of "too many cooks in the kitchen," but the reality is, this type of purposeful transparency makes the operation safer. Now that I am in the position to train residents, I capitalize on every opportunity possible to emphasize the need for transparency in creating narratives. After all, narratives are rooted in clarity, truth telling, and resonance and are buoyed by the character traits discussed in the two prior chapters. Humility, empathy, and pronoia quickly teach a resident that it is never just a surgeon that excels, but a surgical team. After I have finished a case, I often bring the resident in training with me to speak with the family. It is important for the student not only to learn what to do in the operating room, but what to do after the operation. While this habit provides an excellent teaching opportunity, the real motive is to foster transparency. Transparency breeds discomfort because its sole purpose is to expose, but it is that exposure that facilitates a decision to be better or not. When New York State decided to make the morbidity results of its cardiac surgery programs public information, some programs thrived while others initially floundered under such transparency. These programs caved under the pressure to change and become better or shut down. But, after a while, the process of the underperforming programs resulted in better overall outcomes throughout the state. This no-where-to-hide mentality forced these programs to ante up, because it is human nature to behave differently—more humbly and empathetically—when everyone is looking. In 2009, Atul Gawande wrote an article detailing the high costs and degree of unnecessary care that occurred in McAllen, Texas, relative to another town in Texas. The article inspired a scrutiny of the town's medical habits and subsequently served as an impetus for change. When he revisited the town years later, the situation was far better in terms of medical care, but what I was struck by was not so much the changes that were affected by the scrutiny, but that the doctors seemed happier. Doctors are happier when they are adding value.

Exposure is not enough, however. If we only make "numbers" transparent, the programs will respond only to these numbers. Taking the cardiac programs as an example, hard cases may be avoided that would potentially hurt their numbers. This is not what transparency is trying to accomplish. Similarly, if the focus is on patient satisfaction, prioritizing what makes the patients happy, rather than making the patients healthful, may be an unwanted consequence.

We cannot cherry pick transparency. At the risk of overusing idioms, this is an all-or-nothing issue. Just like something can't be "a little freezing" or "slightly closed," transparency means just that—see-through. When I am with a patient, transparency allows me to freely and unapologetically restate numbers, statistics, or other technical information, but for them to truly *see through* is to unabashedly share my purpose, various methods, philosophy, and culture. This aids my narrative. In fact, it is the narrative in and of itself. But as much as a narrative must be transparent, it cannot be one-sided. The final piece comes from the patients. The patients must read and understand the narratives. The patients must take responsibility for understanding. This autonomy completes the process, and is transformative.

Our society is going through a transition. As consumers, aficionados of art, or gatherers of information, we are going from liking what we see to seeing what we like. This is why the consumer and not the provider in medicine will ultimately be in the driver's seat. This is scary to doctors, but when it happens—and it will—doctors will end up happier. Doctors are happy when they create patient autonomy.

A Web of Transparency

This transition from liking what we see to seeing what we like has been be facilitated by the Internet. Marshall McLuhan is credited with the concept that the medium through which a message is disseminated is as important as the actual content of that message. Well, the medium is the message in medicine. This alliterative adaptation of McLuhan's idea suggests that how we communicate about disease has the power to change disease.

This sounds crazy. We know that viruses cause colds and that cigarettes cause lung cancer. Disease is disease and the Internet can't change this can it?

Most of us appreciate the world-changing effect that the printing press, the radio, and the television had on us. Each medium provided a progressively more efficient dissemination of information, which actually changed not only the way that we functioned, but also the way that we started to think. Do you have any doubt that TV shows like *All in The Family* or *Modern Family* have been instrumental in making us more open-minded about racism and homosexuality?

Traditionally, medicine has functioned like TV. Patients were similar to the passive families in their living rooms enjoying and deriving benefit from the content provided. It is similar to listening to your doctor tell you about your disease while you sit passively with your arms on your lap in the office. No doubt this has many positive effects.

Now we have the Internet—the ultimate purveyor of transparency. Not only is it possible to receive information instantly and effortlessly, but unlike TV, the Internet adds two more characteristics to our information gathering. Unlike TV, we can choose both what we want to learn about and when we learn about it. More strikingly distinct from TV, we can also respond to and alter that content. Our interaction with information is thus not only easy and vast (as was made possible with TV), but it is now discretionary and actionable. We have truly become active and partial participants in our own learning.

As the medium of the Internet continues to transform medicine, the way that you will learn about your disease will be similarly altered. You will be able to make a more informed and transparent decision about which doctor you want to see. You will have learned a lot about your health issue prior to going to the doctor's office. By connecting to others with the same symptom or disease, you will not be limited to your doctor's provincial understanding of your disease, its treatment, and how it affects your activities of daily living. Remarkably, you will be able to assume an active role and provide meaningful content about your disease to other sufferers and change the way that those patients and, ultimately, your doctor thinks about your disease.

That's right, this actionable medium will actually allow you to change the disease.

Daniel Pink points out in his book *To Sell Is Human* that our modern connectivity has changed the world from a "buyer beware" mode into a "seller beware" mode (*caveat emptor to caveat venditor*). Anyone selling a product better be trying to sell what is best for the buyer and not best for the seller. This applies to our narratives. Healthcare will be better if our narratives are directed to what is best for the patient. So for doctors, it is *caveat venditor* (seller beware). We need to not only have the knowledge base provided by medical school and the experience of practicing medicine, but we have to become curators of healthcare.

By curator I go to its root which is "taking care of" to depict a different relationship with knowledge. It is not simply the acquisition of knowledge that is important but the contextualizing of that knowledge and the art of sharing that knowledge.

Medicine has lagged behind with regard to this shift because medicine lacks the necessary transparency to put the consumers of healthcare in a position of power. Even if there are currently no numbers to access and no opportunity to get a preview in the operating room, the patient can make a pretty good decision provided he has two things going for him. First, he has spent some time gaining some education in health and in understanding his own expectations and predilections, i.e., he is a patient who has *become a better patient*. Second, he has transparent access to the various available doctors' narratives.

With this in mind, doctors have to understand that our role is changing. Few other businesses can survive without being centered on the customer. In other businesses, the customer can compare price, review other customer satisfaction reports and even sample the merchandise and return it if it is not up to par. This is not really available in medicine.

When a patient comes to see me with a back problem I have already suggested that I need to find the right treatment not only for that particular condition, but for that particular patient with that particular problem. Being a curator adds yet another layer of nuance to this task. I must help the patient not only solve a problem, but help the patient identify the problem. This is the modern essence of expertise.

Daniel Pink refers to this as attunement. He points out that as we become more powerful, we become less attuned. Paradoxically, we gain power by giving up power. In what he calls persuasion jujitsu, using perspective taking, empathy and humility (sound familiar?), we gain, rather than lose, our abilities to be effective doctors.

This is particularly clear to me in my role as department chairman. Consider the plight of a patient who presents to the hospital with a neurosurgical problem. The patient is assigned to the neurosurgeon on call. Shouldn't that patient have transparent access to all of the neurosurgeons that service the hospital? What if the patient needs a procedure and there is another surgeon who has done more of that procedure? Shouldn't the patient at least be aware of such basic information?

As department chairman, I would like to make the process more transparent, but most neurosurgeons feel entitled to care for "their" patient. They have acceptable training, board certification, and more than enough experience. Who am I to judge who is better and how does one even compare surgeons? Providing the patient with another surgeon in the department represents a restriction of trade in the mind of the surgeon on call.

Transparency may ultimately hurt the pocketbook of the surgeon on call, but putting the patient in driver's seat with access to all of the surgeons and their narratives will result in better quality and more satisfaction.

Like a rising tide, transparency floats all boats.

CHAPTER 15

The Narrative and Character

Our narratives arise from our character. They are communicated by transparency. The process of creating our narratives from our character starts with a willingness to scrutinize and modify, rather than reflexively defend, who we are and what we believe. Earlier in the Philosophy section, I outlined the character traits that are essential for this scrutiny, particularly empathy and humility. The stronger the character, the stronger the narrative. So how do we work on our character?

Character is developed through purposeful introspection and then expression. Sounds like a mouthful—introspection and expression—but the idea is to purposefully set aside time to learn and reflect and then to express what we have learned. This expression can be in the form of writing, teaching, mentoring, or best, transparently sharing. The point is that the formal act of expression enhances the act of learning and promotes change when necessary.

Introspection is a concept that seems to be disappearing in our culture. We spend our time on social media or tedious email exchanges. While we feel busy and engaged in these activities, we fail to recognize the lost opportunity for introspection. We end up merely collecting, rather than connecting, the dots.

The real power of our narratives comes after patients and doctors have each developed their own individual narratives. It arises from the doctor-patient relationship. Such a narrative allows for a new consideration of medical expertise. This expertise arises when an expert on the subject matter (the doctor) forms a joint narrative with an expert on the patient (the patient). This is a modern sense of expertise, which is a dynamic, rather than, static state. Gone is the *Encyclopedia Britannica* concept of expertise, with its nominal, arbitrary experts. Enter the Wikipedia type of expertise with its dynamic core defined by an input from many sources, carved out through compromise, rethinking, and real-time correction. Similarly, medical expertise is not what is written in a textbook. Medical expertise is dynamic. It changes as literature is introduced. It is modified or nuanced when the literature doesn't provide a definite answer. It utilizes the patient, who is an expert in what he or she wants and is willing to risk or work for.

The Formation of the Narrative

Mihaly Csikszentmihalyi, in his book *Flow: The Psychology of Optimal Experience*, describes the paradox of work. The paradox of work is that while we feel we can't wait for work to end much of the time, we are, in reality, more fulfilled at work than during our leisure time. He references an experiment in which cell phones were used to randomly interrupt people several times a day. At the time of the interruption, the subjects were asked to document what they were doing and how they felt. It turns out that there is a difference between what we think makes us happy and fulfilled and what actually makes us happy and fulfilled.

Applying this disconnect to the habits of doctors and patients would suggest that a purposeful allotment of time working on their respective narratives of health may seem tedious, but will not only improve our overall health, but increase our happiness and fulfillment.

It will also serve as an antidote to technology. We have a technology paradox as well as a work paradox. We are driven to technology. We know that dopamine is released (the pleasure hormone) when we surf the Internet. And yet, I believe that we are ultimately happier and more fulfilled when we are purposefully resistant to this draw.

Much has been written on the effects of computers on our modern lives. We have become a sitting culture. Children appear to prefer virtual reality to reality. We are struck by images of teenagers sitting together in a room with each on a smartphone surfing the Internet or in "conversation" with friends—some of whom are in the same room. In this context, I am interested in these kids alternatively spending time either purposefully learning alone or when together, in conversation with each other. In a recent experiment, subjects so hated time in solitude that they self-administered electric shocks as a preferable alternative. Solitude becomes an opportunity rather than torture when we have a plan.

I believe that despite our gravitating to the world of the virtual or social media, we actually are happier and more fulfilled when engaged in a different way. Think of our brains in a battle between purposeful engagement and distraction. Engagement refers to a deliberate use of time to learn, reflect and develop our character and philosophy. Distraction allows for the heteronomous control of our actions, habits, and self by business and technology. If we are not deliberate about engagement, however, distraction will always win.

Idle time, like water and air, should be conceptualized as an invaluable commodity. It deserves the same protection as does water and air. This protection must be deliberate, as business and technology will always serve to tarnish it—not out of malevolence, but as a byproduct of their own empowerment.

In medicine there has been a similar move away from engagement. Doctors are caught up in their own routines. We find ourselves doing what is easier rather than what is better for our patients and more fulfilling for us. Rather than learn something new, it is easier to ask for a consult. This leads to passivity. This, too, is the result of our fee-for-service system where doctors try to maximize their volume of patients per allotment of time. The patient is often forced into a role of general contractor in trying to coordinate the various specialists. The pace of medicine doesn't permit effective communication and that renders the patient's experience a piece-meal process.

Patients are similarly victims of distraction over engagement. They are willing to surf the Internet and "shop" for doctors or gain a superficial overview of their condition, but how often do they set aside time to really learn about their condition? The message is that our attention needs to be orchestrated by an intentional design. We need to become choice architects in our attainment of health.

So, how do we use deliberate hard work to create passion in our health? I believe that the process is slightly different for doctors and patients.

For doctors to mitigate the tyrannical changes that business and technology have instilled into medicine they need to create an online persona. This will be further explored in chapter 19. Doctors have always been uncomfortable is such a role. It forces us to place our philosophy and practice in a format that can be scrutinized. It is a transparency that makes us feel vulnerable. On the other hand, it is a phenomenon that has infiltrated most other business worlds and will become part of medicine whether or not we are comfortable with it. I challenge any doctor to conduct an informal poll of his new patients. I guarantee that the majority have done some online research on him.

What is so great about providing philosophy as content on an online platform is that it forces us to read the current literature and remain up-to-date. In addition to reading, it forces us to organize the new material and to synthesize what we have learned with what we already know and what we have uniquely synthesized in the past. Through the process of engagement and putting our thoughts online and making it discoverable, we are not only defining ourselves formally but also transforming ourselves.

Technology may make us partly obsolete, but in producing a unique and philosophical spin on our areas of expertise, we are making ourselves valuable again. Remember that humanity is more important than the hands of a surgeon. I promise that the experience is transformative. An online platform leads to creativity, niche specialization, and satisfaction. Focusing on what the patient wants and needs will make us more empathetic and better doctors—as well as more fulfilled doctors.

Patients, similarly, can benefit from structured, deliberate time spent in the acquisition of health. Patients are subject to the same negative forces of business and technology. There has been recent debate over whether we possess truly autonomous selves, capable of free will. In medicine, this plays out with the obese patient who stops off at McDonald's on his way home. It is easy enough to say that such a decision is the patient's choice. But the convenience and price of the food, along with the care put into optimizing its fat and salt content makes the experience almost irresistible. The crisis we face with our autonomy is not one of free will as much as one of attention. Our attention in pursuit of skills, knowledge, and health habits has been derailed by the deliberate introduction of self-serving distractions used by business for their marketing purposes.

Technology has acted as a co-conspirator by increasing our appetite for distractions. We are increasingly finding pleasure in cyberspace while the dehumanizing part of technology shifts our attention from rewarding but more difficult human interactions to easier and addictive interactions with technology. Perhaps this is epitomized by the recent introduction of the neologism "phubbing," which represents the act of marginally maintaining conversation while tending to one's cell phone. In medicine, a similar process unfolds in the office where doctors simultaneously complete the electronic medical record as they take a medical history or carry on a conversation with the patient.

When patients make the effort to learn about the staples of health like diet and exercise and then make a deliberate strategy to execute their plans, they have the best chance of acquiring health. When patients are faced with disease, they are best served by not simply learning facts about their disease, but trying to understand the new language, the pathophysiology, and the different philosophies of care. When they do all of this, patients will be essentially formulating their narratives, which will become the antidote to the distractions and bait-and-switch diversions. In addition, when patients enter online discussions of their disease they contribute to the understanding of the disease. In this manner they become transformative agents of change as discussed in a previous chapter.

The need to develop our narrative is now greater than ever as we sit on the forefront of a deluge of data that will come from increased genome sequencing and patient-driven self-monitoring of pulse, daily steps taken, blood pressure, blood glucose and many other soon to be measurable components of health. This data will be effortlessly acquired and owned by the patient due to the improvement in computing power that we now have available. It will empower our narratives. Without narratives, it will be a potential source of more medicalization—a disaster.

PART IV

THE PRESCRIPTION

Inside You'll Find:

I have learned not only the importance of *conveying* a genuine interest in my patient and his or her condition, but that I must also *have* an interest.

How such interest is developed, articulated, executed, and exchanged is the purpose of The Prescription. It is the responsibility of both the patient and the doctor not only to have a dialogue and narrative with themselves about their own value systems, but also to direct the introspective work they do toward an active and engaged communication with one another. As in any relationship, individuals who truly understand themselves, are secure with how they feel, and are honest about what they want, make more successful partners. The Me in Medicine's intent is to forge and sustain successful partnerships, and therefore relies on the practice of distinct narratives, which begins our journey into the Prescription.

CHAPTER 16

The Narrative as an Approach to Back Pain

Back pain requires a deliberate, intentional, and plodding fix. My first book, *The End of Back Pain,* advocates for an alternative, slow and steady, approach to treatment, which includes education and progressive exercise. My personal brand of treatment looks to diminish the frequency, duration, and intensity of the invariable episodes of back pain. This slower fix looks to build back health rather than eliminate pain because this is what I have found, in my twenty plus years as a neurosurgeon, to work the best.

Building back health requires both a commitment to education and a sustained program of exercise. Exercise provides a method of fundamentally changing your back. It harnesses your body's innate capacity to adapt positively to stress. A combination of aerobic conditioning and core strengthening works best. There is a pervasive idea that doing abdominal work will help back pain. This is partially correct, but abdominal work alone is not sufficient. Our core is comprised of much more than our abdominal muscles. The core is a circumferential group of connected muscles that includes the abdominal muscles, but also includes back muscles called the multifidus muscles. These muscles are essential to core strengthening. In the *End of Back Pain,* I focus on this part of the core that is usually overlooked. I refer to it as the hidden core. Your hidden core is the most important aspect and least utilized aspect of core strengthening. I have found that prioritizing these back muscles is most effective in promoting back health.

If I were to rely on narratives to help my back-pain patients adopt my philosophy as their own, as opposed to seeking surgery, I would contextualize back pain with an analogy of cardiac disease. A fifty-something who suffers a minor heart attack will likely have two responses. The first is the idea that he has been dealt a bad heart and should seek medications or surgery to mitigate such bad fortune (victim mentality). The second, alternative response is for the patient to fundamentally change the caliber and function of his coronary arteries through intense and sustained exercise and dietary intervention.

Obviously, the second response is a slow fix, but the more effective one, as the lifestyle changes will strengthen and protect the heart after the attack, but strengthen the entire body over time. As with the heart, the exercises for back health represent the most important part of the slow fix, and the patients whom I have helped treat their back pain with lifestyle changes not only have better backs but also better overall health and strength. When patients improve their strength and fitness, their back feel better, but they also sleep better, enjoy better moods, and are less anxious. The slow fix improves overall health as it improves back health.

Furthering my narrative, I would include storytelling, such as retelling one of my favorite parables of the tortoise and the hare. It is obvious that the faster animal should win the race. In fact, if the hare were to take the race seriously, he would undoubtedly win. With this in mind, we should aspire to be the hare. But this assumption is wrong. We fail to see the real strength of the tortoise, which is not only its dogged perseverance and focus, but also its ability to resist being saddled by convictions and assumptions and to look beyond obvious concepts. Slow *can* win the race.

I tell my patients with back pain that they need to start their exercises while still in some pain. You could imagine some of the crazy looks I get. I tell them that letting "pain be your guide" is potentially limiting, and thus, potentially a harmful rule of thumb.

Teaching them to embrace shades of gray and to attempt some paradoxes, I tell patients to move even if moving is painful. Now that I have included in my narrative anecdotes and storytelling, I finalize our conversation with personal empathy, saying that I realize this advice is unsettling and counterintuitive, but as back pain sufferer myself, I know it can lead to breakthroughs in pain relief. It is the tortoise, and not the hare, who is willing to take that advice and, it is the tortoise, and not the hare, who prevails.

As we are often our own worst enemies is life, the same is true in confronting back pain. Accepting conventional wisdom can often lead you down a longer path of suffering with unsatisfactory results. Challenging assumptions, getting educated and taking charge of back health is the safest and surest path to a more pain free existence.

In this book, I continue on the path of alternative and holistic treatments by introducing the utilization of narratives for the treatment of back pain. Providing narratives is so much more than just talking. Narratives circumvent the status quo of treatment, making it far-reaching enough to engage patients and doctors in eight important ways.

1. **Place the patient in the driver's seat.** This will counter the most dangerous force in the treatment of back pain: The treatment rendered depends mostly on where the patient chooses to go for help rather than what is actually wrong. We must place the patient above our own self-interests.

2. **Substitute the emotion of equanimity for panic.** Teach the patient to view back pain as a part of life, like the common cold or headache rather, than the consequence of an injury. Obviously, there is a small subsection of back pain that requires the full force and capabilities of the medical system, but that is the minority of back pain pursued only in limited circumstances.

3. **Promote education.** Education is an independent determinant of health and the patient has to be pushed to spend some energy and time to learn. Perhaps the most important educational goal is outing the false assumptions about treating back pain.

4. **Foster self-efficacy.** Substitute the adaptable mindset for the vulnerable mindset. Having the confidence to take on a problem, both learning about it and taking responsibility for its treatment is another independent enabler in health. The secret to success in back pain is to attain independence from pain medication, therapists, surgeons, etc.

5. **Redirect the patient's energy.** The actual search for a definite diagnosis or easy solution, while reasonable at first, is often counterproductive and exhausting. At some point, a redirection of energy toward coping and returning to daily activities can be a healing mechanism in and of itself. Patients are often unaware of how much energy they are using to either obtain an answer or look for a solution. At some point, that energy is better spent in finding ways to cope with the pain.

6. **Expose biases.** Patients (and doctors) are terribly flawed in their decision processes. Understanding our biases makes us better decision makers. This enlightenment also frees the patient from the tyranny of the well-intentioned and anecdotally based advice from family and friends.

7. **Use the three wonderfully refreshing words: "I don't know."** Some of your patients will be put off by your apparent deficiency, but these words, more than not, reflect the truth and are an important part of communication and treatment.

8. **Ignite the placebo effect.** This is the doctor's greatest strength. Doctors have the capacity not only to make patients feel better,

but be better. Our words do more than soothe, they heal. Our bodies are designed to heal themselves. The role of doctor has been enhanced by technology and knowledge, but the doctor's humanity along with an ability to teach, contextualize, and empathize remains the most powerful instrument of change in our health system.

Patient narratives can similarly circumvent the status quo of treatment. Many of the above narratives can be applied by the patients. I would also offer the following patient-specific narratives in addition

1. **Assume responsibility of care coordinator.** Although it is easy to presume that the doctor will be thinking more about your problem when you leave, this is unlikely. Follow up on results and coordination between specialists are your responsibility.

2. **Don't be overly swayed by a confident doctor.** Surgeons are particularly guilty of the state, "never in doubt, often wrong." You should receive all advice with some healthy skepticism.

3. **Listen with an open mind.** It is important to remember that your presumptions may interfere with what you can learn. While it is typically the doctor that needs to listen better, the patient is similarly afflicted by a closed mind.

4. **Collect all of your office notes, lab reports, and test results.** One day this will be stored on your smartphone. Don't expect this gathering to occur naturally. It is your job.

5. **Ask to have the natural history outlined when a treatment is offered.** Patients have a tendency to focus on the pros and cons of treatment, but forget to contrast that with the pros and cons of doing nothing.

6. **Become a writer.** Nothing will solidify what you have learned at the office visit more than writing a synopsis of not only what the doctor said, but your thoughts as well. Articulating what you have experienced will also help you to figure out what to do next.

CHAPTER 17

The Narrative of the Future

When it comes to understanding narrative medicine, this idea of tension is critical, as it is my experience that the exploration, creation, and communication of one's narrative requires tension to occur, first within oneself, and then between doctor and patient. By tension I mean the verb form, which is defined as "to apply a force to (something) that tends to *stretch* it [emphasis mine]."

In other words, out of chaos comes progress in the form of the expansion of our understanding of our humanity and our necessary connection to one another, as practitioners and patients.

The same is true in narrative medicine. There are three very separate, yet interdependent stories occurring in the same setting, centered on the same theme, but with varying viewpoints necessary to the composition and success of the story itself: the doctor's narrative, the patient's narrative, and the doctor-patient narrative. Much of this book has focused on the importance and formation of narratives by both doctors and patients. A transformative event arises when these individually developed narratives come together in a unique doctor-patient narrative.

We must rustle our own feathers, acknowledge our faults and bad habits and assumptions, and get real about what we want, what we value, and how we want to proceed in our own healthcare, from the perspective of the providers and patients. For doctors, this means going to the darkest places, where the undesirable traits that are responsible for the "problems" in healthcare exist: hubris, misdirection, and fear of failure. For patients, their exploration into their psyche includes the foibles of decision-making, overestimating the role of the paternalistic doctor, and underestimating their own potential to learn and gain autonomy and self-efficacy. Coming to terms with these tensions, the things that threaten us from becoming ourselves, helps us get closer to the narratives that empower us.

The Doctor's Narrative

The idea of the post-surgical narrative came to me after the horrific loss of a partner who died in a plane crash. We had worked together for more than ten years. When it was time to give his eulogy, I insisted on being the one to deliver it. Of the many stories that went through my mind, I particularly remembered accompanying him as he spoke with a patient's family after a difficult operation on the brain. What I so vividly remember was that despite being given the opportunity to alter some of the more difficult aspects of the case, he chose to be direct—even to the point where it undermined his own performance.

I expected the family to be critical of him or to lose faith in him, but what I saw was unadulterated appreciation. I was so moved by this gesture of authenticity, of my partner's connection, adherence to, and credence to his own value system. I reflected on the situation and etched into my brain—and my heart—a promise that I would forever handle the surgical narrative as my partner had that day.

Many doctors will reminisce about the good old days when they had the time, the patience, the inclination, the support, and the subsidies that enabled them to sit with and invest in their patients and their families on a deep level. Even the vernacular we use to describe such a doctor has changed from "family doctor" to one that is "primary," meaning the doctor isn't necessarily a go-to, but the first in the long line of protocol.

You may have been one of the many people who have been restlessly sitting in the surgical waiting room while your loved one is undergoing an operation. Suddenly you are wrested from your pensive state as the surgeon is standing in front of you. You have so many questions, but what you *really* need to know is whether everything went as planned. The surgeon who has done the hard work of creating his or her own narratives will already know this and be empathetic, and thus should have a narrative that is first and foremost open-minded and truthful.

While it is tempting to edit the events of the case to protect myself or to impress the family, transmitting exactly what I feel and believe is an honor and an opportunity for connection.

My Not-So-*Me*-in-Medicine Moment

Years ago, I was doing an emergency operation at night in a small private hospital. The patient had a hemorrhage in the brain that required evacuation. I was on call and buckled down knowing that I would be actively involved in the procedure for several hours.

When these events occur at night, it is not uncommon to spend a couple of hours alone with the surgical scrub tech working together to get the task done. Depending on the difficulty of the procedure, we can work in atmospheres of near silence to a highly animated room with music playing boldly in the background.

This particular night was relatively mellow and the surgical scrub tech and I were moving along with light conversation when he politely asked me, "Can I give you some constructive feed-back?" He was a very overqualified scrub tech, as he had been a surgeon in Poland and had not been able to transfer his degree to America when he was forced to leave his country.

"Sure," I said, expecting to hear something related to the surgery. "You were an asshole today."

I looked up briefly and let him continue, describing the way that I had treated the circulating nurse during the early part of the case. Although he acknowledged that the nurse had not performed adequately during previous cases and that he understood my frustration with her, the scrub tech aptly pointed out that during this particular evening she had done nothing wrong, and yet, I had been mean to her. In fact, she had left the room in tears and was now replaced by a different nurse. All of this had transpired without my knowledge.

I continued to work quietly, the word asshole still looming in the air, while I considered the evening and my behavior. I had, in fact, attacked the nurse for no good reason. In retrospect, over the previous several times that we had worked together, I had become increasingly more impatient with her. I also remembered that during my training, one of my mentors would ceaselessly pick on several nurses that he didn't care for. As a resident, I remember thinking that I would remember this behavior as a model for what *not* to do. Now, I found myself in the role of bully. Deplorable.

When you finish your residency and become an attending physician, nothing really changes and yet everything is different. You continue to do what you have done for the past several years, but the way that you are treated is not the same. Suddenly all decisions are deferred to you. "What temperature do you want the room?" or "What music would you like on?" It must be like the military where there is a ranking that makes the various relationships unequivocally defined. When one goes from bottom rung to top dog, it is easy to slip into the role of a bully. It happens insidiously and even when one has previously vowed never to act like that.

After several more minutes of considering that my scrub tech thought I was an asshole, I excused myself from the patient for a moment and sought out the nurse. I gave her a sincere apology and then returned to finish what I started.

When a friend walks into a room with a piece of food visible on his tooth, do you let him know—even if it is awkward? I hope so. When people slip into undesirable states of behavior that they may not be aware of, is it appropriate to point it out?

"Thank you," I said to my surgical scrub tech. "Thank you for slapping me in the face. I needed that."

Solving Problems with Doctor Narratives

"The wheel is come full circle," said Edmund in Shakespeare's *King Lear*. However, completing a cycle or returning to its beginnings doesn't have to mean facing an ill fate, as when Edgar sought his revenge on Edmund. In putting the Me in Medicine, we use narratives to address the problems of our medical system, which were identified and defined at the beginning this book. Now, as we come full circle in our discussion, the prescription of narratives can be tailored and utilized to turn an ill fate into action and true change, miles away from the problems we face right now.

Narrating the Problem of the Need for Diagnosis and Disease

In chapter 1, I introduced you to John, who had been diagnosed with fibromyalgia, but had come to see me because of a new pain. On heels of his fibromyalgia diagnosis John couldn't help but assume his pain was related. No doubt, if John had not been given such a diagnosis, this correlation would not have played a part in John's interpretation of the pain. He figured that if the pain was not related, then something new and unrelated had occurred. If his pain was something new, it must be an injury or something broken. John came to this conclusion because, in his mind, all pain has a cause and resolution of the pain requires treatment or a fixing of that cause. This is the power of personal perception at work—his outlook literally made him jump to a conclusion.

This scenario is an example of the problem of the need for disease and diagnosis, as described in Part I. But what if John had spent a little time learning about pain? What if he had learned that back pain is common and that the cause is often not determinable? What if he knew that back pain is like a headache; it comes from time to time and then goes away. In that setting, he would not have had the same reaction to the pain. He would have had faith in his body's capacity to resolve the pain. Not only would he have a different outlook, but also, he would have experienced less pain because of that different outlook.

How would John have learned about the complexities of pain? He didn't complete four years of medical school. He doesn't have the confidence to buy a book on pain. There is an Internet available to John. He can sit in his kitchen and not only have access to a variety of articles on pain, but to many doctors and other providers who have written perspectives on how to treat pain and how to deal with pain. John's job is not to find the correct approach, because there is no correct approach. There are many points of view. John's job is to read with an open mind and find a point of view that resonates with his own sensibilities, to do his own contextualizing. John's job is to not be intimidated by the subject matter and to spend some time trying to learn and analyze what seems right to him. John must have a healthy skepticism of the treatments offered him.

When I met with John to work out his problem together, I was initially frustrated. Each time I brought up a possible path, he was resistant: "I tried that already" or "Physical therapy never works." I realized that there were two obstacles in the way. First, John was saddled by his own convictions, many of which were instilled by friends and families unabashedly offering solutions without any knowledge. They are fueled by anecdotes. In this case, I challenged

John on the sources of his convictions and tried to show him how faulty anecdotes of other people's conditions or experiences could be, especially when they are stories of friends of friends of friends. When pressed, John realized that what he had been hearing was speculation. As he was made aware of the limitations of thinking in anecdotes, he became more willing to consider the possibility of treatments. The second obstacle that needed to be overcome was mine. I had been focusing on John being stubborn, while I had failed to understand that much of his stubbornness was generated from fear. This became apparent through our dialogue. Rather than push my agenda, I forced myself to listen to John. John was afraid to come off his pain medication. This is not unusual in patients who have been taking pain medications chronically. Separating the plan to get John off his pain medications from the plan for physical therapy helped John not to reject all treatment. By summoning up my compassion, I was able to meet John where he was and work in tandem with the pace he felt most comfortable with.

Finally, John and I sat down and talked about fibromyalgia. He came to understand the meaning of the chameleon effect. I gave him examples of how I had fallen prey to the chameleon effect— how I had arrogantly and hypocritically told patients to exercise while I hesitated to exercise my body when I learned of my own herniated disc. We spent a good deal of time discussing that it is more useful to view the human body as adaptable rather than vulnerable. He had assumed that exercise would serve to potentially exacerbate his pain rather than to cause an adaptation and serve as a protector. I shared with John how strong my instinct had been that exercise would exacerbate my condition. I shared that each time I suffer an exacerbation of back pain it requires a "leap of faith" to restart activities as there is always an underlying fear that "maybe this time something really is wrong."

Six months later John was much better. He had forced himself to do what he presumed would increase his pain. Some of his activities did make him feel worse, but he used equanimity, and not panic, to face these setbacks. Some of the activities made him feel better—something that he hadn't expected. When I asked him what made him better, John provided a most curious response, "I'm not sure if I am better or whether I have just learned to live with the pain."

My narrative had led him to the reality that learning to live with back pain is often the same as being better.

Narrating the Problem of the Provider on the Pedestal

Alexis was the patient who had an MRI which showed a herniated disc and was sent to physical therapy. She was led from one provider to the next due to a rabbit hole of an MRI report, which had shown a herniated disc. Her narrative was characterized by two flaws: "doctor knows best" and that the herniated disc was the cause of her pain.

Like John, Alexis needed to be disabused of these convictions. I explained to her that the herniated disc might not be the cause of her pain. I told her that if I arbitrarily took a bunch of people off the street who experienced no back pain, MRIs would reveal a large percentage of these asymptomatic people to have herniated discs. The herniated disc might mean nothing in her case because it is often present and not painful and I explained to Alexis that as a fellow back pain sufferer and as a surgeon, *that* I had even symptomatic herniated discs heal on their own. Unabashedly I invited Alexis into the private world of medicalization, explaining to her how and why providers lean on diagnosing people with herniated discs. I could see she was enlightened and refreshed by my honesty when I told her that diagnosis was used to explain her pain and, thus, wrap up her office visit. It was used as a rationale for treatment by the physical therapists. It served the providers—the one's that she had put on a pedestal—and not her. My narrative was used to help disillusion Alexis.

Once Alexis realized that her disc herniation didn't need to be fixed and was unlikely to be the cause of her pain, she started to get better. The most important lesson for Alexis was that she must serve in an autonomous role. She came to understand that education is an independent enabler of health.

Most patients have assumed a passive role in their quest for health and treatment of disease. They have been prey to the ubiquitous marketing of fast food, quick fixes, and Big Pharma. They have followed the self-serving script written by the medical providers, which reads: When you get a disease, you *need us* to get you better. Medicine has become formidable and certainly does help many patients get better, but as we have seen, it also carries a risk of harm as well. The autonomous patient armed with self-efficacy is better positioned to avoid treatment that has no merit— even when advocated for by those on a pedestal. The autonomous patient views the concept *"need us"* as problematic.

And at the end of the day, even if the patient holds true to their conviction that they need me to help them, I know I have given them all the facts, all the lenses, and the truth, and that is really all I can do to stay true to my character.

Narrating the Problem of Fee-for-Service Medicine

Remember Adam? He was the patient contemplating spinal surgery out of desperation. He not only had to worry about a surgery that would be unpredictable in terms of success, but he had to worry about his insurance company approving the surgery in the event that he was willing to undergo the risk.

While it was tempting to pit Adam against the insurance company and its evil desire to save money, this would only serve as a distraction from the difficult decision of whether or not to have surgery. I also had to consider my own temptation. If I explained to Adam that the risk was his to decide and he ended up disappointed after surgery, I could hide behind my preoperative disclaimers and walk away with a clear conscious and more money in my bank account.

Would I have gone through such a surgery if I felt what Adam felt? Of course, one can never know what a patient feels, but I do know that I wouldn't undergo a surgery with such bad odds. My narrative became focused on making sure that Adam understood the most likely postoperative course versus the possibility of relief of his pain. I have learned over the years that desperate patients tend to hear what they want (a potential upside) and not what is most likely to occur (disappointment). I understood that it was Adam's decision to make, but I needed to make sure that he saw both sides of the future. If I hadn't passed on what I have witnessed over the years I have provided surgery, I wouldn't be true to my narrative.

Adam ultimately chose to have surgery. His gains were minimal. Strangely enough, he had no regrets. He found it easier to deal with the pain once he felt that he had done everything possible. That kind of peace of mind, even if it is not peace from pain, is what is of utmost importance to me and is what drives my narrative.

Narrating the Problem of Overtreatment

I am called to see a patient with a catastrophic brain hemorrhage. The patient was in a motor vehicle accident and has sustained trauma to the brain. A CT scan shows brain swelling intermixed with hemorrhage. I have examined the patient and immediately understand that this is not a survivable injury. Interestingly, I know this within seconds of seeing the patient and the CT scan.

My mind is not focused on survival statistics for this type of injury. I am not worried that I may be "missing" something on the exam or CT scan. I am focused on my impending interaction with the family. The issue here is no longer the patient, for what has happened cannot be undone or remedied.

How I interact with the family, however, has the potential to make this terrible situation more tolerable. It has the potential to lead them to a sensible decision regarding treatment. It has the potential to make them feel slightly better by providing a different perspective, a small silver lining to a large gray cloud.

The encounter also has the potential to make things worse. I could create disagreement among the family members. I could present a view that not only does not resonate with the family's sensibilities, but actually antagonizes them. Moreover, I will not be able to know how they are reacting until I am well into our conversation.

Again, the art of communication and the need for the proper narrative is imperative. In this case, I am not only trying to lessen their pain, but to convey that "doing something" is not always better than not doing something.

In this case, the family is large. It is immediately obvious that they are hysterical. My instincts tell me that they need someone who is calm. I start off by recounting what has happened and with a description (that they can understand) of how their loved one is doing now.

My logical next step is to go directly into prognosis, but I have learned that I am better off not pushing this, but rather answering this question only when asked. Most families have a way of letting me know what they are ready to hear and when. If the family is ready to take on the prognosis, they will typically ask the question explicitly.

In this case the question is asked explicitly and hysterically. Because the family is large, some are asking for prognosis while others are urging that I not be interrupted. This is a typical situation as some will want to hear everything while others prefer that I decide what is appropriate to discuss—the typical seesaw in medicine between the paternalistic doctor and the autonomous patient or family.

I know that I will need to discuss prognosis because it is loudly and directly asked of me, and yet, I also know that I will be giving other members of the family more information than they want or are capable of processing. I am careful to use eye contact with each of the family members. I also know that I cannot equivocate, as a mixed message will create more harm than good.

Early in my career when dealing with a situation where a patient was on a ventilator but had no brain function, I made the mistake of presenting the situation as the "family's choice." The fact was that the patient was already dead, but I was intimidated by the sheer amount of family emotion and told them that we would not rush them and would allow them to decide on whether the ventilator would be disconnected. My lack of direction ultimately necessitated an intervention from the hospital ethics committee and other more senior physician involvement. I learned after this that the truth must be explicitly stated, as ambiguity can create unnecessary pain for the family.

Back to the case at hand, I continue to tell the family that their loved one has suffered an irreversible injury to the brain and that no treatment can reverse the current situation. There is more hysteria. I feel their pain, but I must remain calm. As much as they may appreciate empathy from me in the form of emotion, what they need more at this moment is calm and reason.

I am asked, "Are you sure?" I reply that I am with a mustered authority. I am asked "Why?," but I don't answer. There is no answer to this question, which is more of a declaration than a question. I give the family time to digest the information and interact with each other. Invariably, some member of the family will emerge as the spokesperson. In this case there is more than one and it appears that they do not agree on what direction we should go.

Some family members want everything done while others what has happened and are focused on not letting the patient suffer.

Even though part of my mind goes to the statistics about much money we waste in end-of-life care, I cannot allow those facts to interfere with my relationship with this family. I have to remain focused on shepherding them through this difficult time.

Over the years, I have been in this situation numerous times. Most families, if they have regrets, will regret that they pushed for "getting everything done." It is easy to conclude this in retrospect and because families typically don't have previous experience, they tend to lack this perspective when making their decision. This is where I can be helpful. I gently let the family know that many families have the instinct to not let go and to preserve life, but later regret that decision when their loved one persists in a chronic vegetative state. It is important for the family to have this added perspective as they are unlikely to incorporate it into their decision.

As the conversation continues, the questions become more directed and appropriate. I have managed to quell the emotional component for the time being and have focused the family on the practical decision-making that is necessary.

I recognize that the patient is already dead, but death has many meanings for many different people. From my neurologically oriented perspective, the patient has died. I recognize that I have a particularly opinionated idea of death. For me, losing what makes us uniquely human is to be dead. Our ability to plan, worry, joke, think, etc., is what we are. Being able to open our eyes, have our hearts beat, and initiate breaths is not enough, but I know that I do not have the right to impose my perspective on others. In these discussions, however, I have learned that sharing my beliefs with the understanding that they are merely one man's opinion is helpful. It is also often helpful for me to offer what I would do if this were my loved one. I let them know. Articulating these ideas is helpful because they are often already in the family's mind, but suppressed because they seem so harsh. When another human being shares them as natural and appropriate feelings, they may emerge.

Since death for this patient is either already here, or at least imminent, I raise the subject of organ donation. The organ donation crew have made it clear to hospital staff that our responsibility is only to ask for permission that the family meet with them. The organ donation caseworkers are highly trained on how to broach the subject. It is hard for me to relinquish this duty as I feel it is part of my responsibility, but I abide by what I have been asked and let the family know that speaking with the organ donor organization is an option.

It is now time to walk away. All families need time on their own to allow the family dynamic to further unfold. I give them some time and let them know how to contact me in the event they have more questions. Inevitably they do and so I don't go too far from the hospital.

An hour or so later the family calls and lets me know that they have decided to speak with the organ donor organization and that they understand that there is nothing else to do. They thank me for my help. It always amazes me that even in such distress most families can acknowledge their appreciation for my facilitation of the process. I leave with two thoughts. The first is that I have made the best of a terrible situation. They have avoided a prolonged situation with a similar ending. Secondly, I ruminate over what I would do in their situation? Empathy is a critical part of communication and because I have chosen to let it, it floods over me now that I have done my job.

Throughout this book there has been in the foreground my own careful exploration of who should be making decisions— the paternalistic doctor or the autonomous patient. In chapter 6, I went as far as to show how we don't need to choose. I engaged in thoughtful, compassionate, transparent, and honest, one-on-one narrative with the family I just spoke of and, in the end, I am reassured that the decision was all of theirs, just made in cooperation with a doctor.

This story could have turned out very differently. I could have suggested that "it can't hurt to try." The family may have taken a different tack in that case. I found myself with a unique opportunity. The way that I guided the family was critical to not only to the patient in distress, but also to the large family. I had the opportunity to positively shape their interpretation of the event and ease their pain. Sometimes, less is more.

Narrating the Problem of Technology

Over the past several years there has been a proliferation in electronic medical records. This technology will undoubtedly bring some very positive changes. As electronic medical records become more ubiquitous, user-friendlier, and more shareable, there will be a surplus of data that will be fodder for intellectual and creative progress. In addition, the use of biosensors connected to our smartphones for personal monitoring will provide additional data in an unprecedented quantity. As this data becomes available it will be analyzed by increasingly powerful computers that will, in turn, generate enormous numbers of correlations and opportunities to better understand our disease processes.

We should not adopt an Orwellian sense of hopelessness in response to the inevitable rising capabilities of the computer, but rather adopt one of relief. The computer's capacity to assist the physician with diagnoses and treatment selection and interpretation of images leaves the physician with more time to act in a humane fashion—as an interpreter, contextualizer, or ombudsman. After so much progress, we are brought back to the role of the doctor making house calls, who long ago didn't have much to offer from the tools in his black bag in terms of technological advances and knowledge, but made it his business to provide support and comfort. Now, with so much more to offer through technology, doctors are freer to take on this essential role, but in addition, we will need to supply our unique narratives, which we have acquired from doctoring. This is how we will be distinguished in a world where our traditional role is slowly usurped by computers. Patients will similarly have to supply their own narratives to protect their individuality. The fullness of the patient narrative, that which includes personal implications, assumptions that are tied to life experience or cultural bias and other emotional states is made generic by a watered-down version that appears in the medical chart. The new story is re-shaped by a vernacular that conforms to models of disease, treatment, and reimbursement.

The advent of electronic medical records (EMR) serves to further alienate the patient from his or her story. The narrative in medicine needs to go both ways. The patient needs to tell his story and the healthcare provider needs to listen to that story, but what is often lost is the second side of this coin.

This increase in automation will provide time to enjoy and encourage a genuine and helpful exchange. The opportunity here is to use the time to exercise our humanity. It is important to remember that computers can't think nor display insight, humility, empathy and many other human qualities that are often helpful in ambiguous situations or situations that are fickle or changing.

We can use our distinct human capabilities to not only construct a narrative arc regarding how a patient got to where he or she is, but to forecast a narrative regarding the future. I have no doubt that computers will replace humans in formulating differential diagnoses, determining the most appropriate tests to order, and even in reading X-rays. At some point, computers may replace surgeons in the operating room. What a computer has great difficulty with is predicting the future, which depends on interpretation of processes that are distinctly human. It is very easy for a computer to tell us who was president of our country in a certain year, but very difficult to predict whom our next president will be.

Pierre-Simon Laplace, the French mathematician, suggested that if we know every detail about a certain current situation, we could predict the future. This optimism arises from elaborate theories that are constructed as to why certain events occur. Actions bring about complicated reactions making the future effects non-linear and very difficult to predict—particularly by a computer. Humans can incorporate intangibles, moods, and instincts into the narrative arcs of the future. While we will never be perfect forecasters, we can become better. This requires practice and scrutiny of our previous predictions. Medicine is replete with sophisticated predictions and bereft of retrospective scrutiny of those predictions. Holding one's predictions accountable and being self-critical leads to improved forecasting. The time created by technology will allow for this pursuit.

Narrating the Problem of Pain

You bend over to pick up the garbage, which weighs only three pounds, and you feel a click or a tiny bit of heat in your back. An hour later you are incapacitated. You can't straighten up, you need help getting out of bed. *Something really bad just happened*, you think.

We are wired to react to pain. Primitive man needed to be alerted when a creature was gnawing at his foot. While this natural tendency is understandable, consider the possibility that sometimes we take it too far.

I have been besieged by back spasms many times. I know that they typically represent a protective, albeit painful, reaction to what is likely a very trivial underlying problem. Nonetheless, my initial reaction is panic. *Maybe something really bad is going on this time.*

This is where I employ my narrative. I have vetted out this situation already. I know that spasms often can be severe and yet, represent only a minor underlying pathology. I know that it will go away in a few days. This control of emotion allows me to let the panic slip away and invite more rational behavior. I don't run to the doctor as this is time-consuming, expensive, and ineffective.

I have addressed this predicament of my innate need to impulsively react to pain with a narrative instead of a treatment. In this case my narrative is both an understanding of the natural history of my predicament and a commitment to a specific emotional response (equanimity). I don't need to know why my back is consumed with spasm. My narrative doesn't initially seek a diagnosis. My narrative views the human body as more adaptive than vulnerable.

CHAPTER 18

The Office Visit of the Future

In the Promise section I talked about office visits of the future. The patient will be armed with knowledge of his genome, proteome, metabolite, exposome, and microbiome, but three important things need to be present in the office visit of the future: transparency, contextualization, and new mental models and habits.

Transparency

Our narratives should be transparently accessible to patients on the Internet. As a surgeon, the patient should have access to how often I perform a particular procedure. The patient should also have access to my interpretation of the science and practice of medicine. With such transparency, the method of referrals will be transformed. The patient will no longer be held hostage to his doctor's referral patterns, which may consist of sending patients to another doctor who is a friend or, worse, to one that will return the favor. The patient may, alternatively, autonomously sample the appropriate specialists and pick one that resonates.

Contextualization

Narrative medicine requires a process of contextualizing. As a surgeon who deals with patients who are experiencing back pain, before discussing treatments, it is essential that I contextualize the back pain. Patients must understand that back pain is part of life for many—most—patients. Treatment cannot be conceptualized as eliminating back pain. It may help but part of treatment is getting the patient to understand that some of the responsibility lies with the patient. The patient must accept back pain and put some energy into coping with back pain. The idea of "cure" is misleading and undermining.

Narrative medicine involves transparency of thoughts between doctor and patient. A common scenario that plays out in the office is a patient telling me that he has a "high tolerance of pain." What is meant to convey toughness to me actually backfires. Most spine surgeons immediately interpret such a claim as a warning sign. "This patient is going to be a problem. He will likely complain more of pain than the average patient." I suspect that the reason for this apparent paradox is that such an affirmation arises from the patient's need to convince himself of his superior tolerance because he is struggling with pain. The fascinating idea here is that by communicating this paradox with patients, it helps them alter their self-perceptions and actually experience less pain. The idea is that the capacity of the doctor to contextualize pain can actually affect the amount of pain, as we discussed in chapter 6.

The office visit of the future will be directed to the attainment of health. What is health anyway? The World Health Organization published its definition of health more than fifty years ago as a state of complete physical, mental, and social wellbeing and not merely the absence of disease or infirmity. Most of us rarely feel like we are in a state of complete physical, mental and social wellbeing. Should we thus conclude that we are not healthy? Of course not. The usefulness of the definition is, first, in understanding that health is not simply the absence of disease. Health is something to actively pursue and acquire. Second, understanding the social aspect of health is critical. The social determinants of health are the unique environments in which people grew up in and currently work and live in. This takes into account an individual's social status, family life, income, upbringing and allows for the presumptions and convictions that come along with it. The responsibility of the patient is thus not only to be medically educated, but to recognize that his or her attainment of health is saddled as much by the presumptions he or she has acquired or the job and job satisfaction he or she has than the specific gene pool he or she was born into.

This is a provocative idea. We have traditionally looked at health as a default state that occurs if there is no disease. Looking at health as attainable through our own actions is the future of medicine. Our first foray into autonomy was preventative medicine. The idea of identifying what we are at risk for, or in the early stages of would potentially offer more effective treatment. We spent billions of dollars sequencing the human genome with the hope that this would unlock the key to the preventative treatment of disease. If each of us would have the opportunity to cheaply sequence our DNA, we would identify what we are at risk for and then try to prevent it.

What's the point of knowing our DNA if we are either cursed or blessed by what we find and have no means to affect destiny? It turns out that we do have the capacity to affect change—not by preventing what we are destined for but by changing our destiny.

There has been much written on the nature versus nurture dilemma. The burgeoning field of epigenetics provides the scientific basis for the answer to the question nature versus nurture— it is both. Nature is the genome that we have been given by our parents. Epigenetics is the role that our lifestyle and environment play in the expression of our genome. It is the nurture. It is the process whereby we change our DNA through our own actions. This change is largely not by changing the DNA itself, but in changing the way our DNA is expressed. This is accomplished by the part of the genome long thought to be "junk" DNA, called "dark matter." Dark matter is the name given to the 98 percent of the human genome that is not involved with protein coding. We now believe

that this part of the DNA codes for RNA, which through topolog-
ical interactions, chemical reactions, and alteration of 3-D configu-
rations can affect, not the DNA, but the way the DNA is expressed.
Traditional ideas of genetics that date back to Mendel and Darwin
have to be reconsidered. Survival of the fittest suggested that evolution proceeded slowly based on the survival advantage of a particular gene expression. Epigenetics suggests that not only can we
alter the expression of our DNA without environment or lifestyle,
but also that we can actually change the DNA. This radical idea
comes from looking at women who experience their pregnancy
during times of extreme stress or in extreme hunger. The babies
who were born out of these situations demonstrate an increased
stress response or tendency to store food. In other words, it is possible that this more rapid evolution occurred not from survival of
the fittest, but from epigenetic alteration of the genes.

Exercise is a great example of the potential of epigenetics to
alter our health. Exercise not only makes us stronger and fitter,
but it changes the expression of our DNA. Control of the DNA
expression is a burgeoning field. Our microbiome, which is the
billions of bacteria that live symbiotically inside and outside of us
can alter gene expression. There is reason to believe that a healthy
lifestyle can lengthen our telomeres, which are the protective ends
of our chromosomes. Shortening of the telomeres and the subsequent vulnerability of our genes to undergo mutations during
division is one of the determinants of aging. This is a method
by which lifestyle can increase longevity. There is even a field
of behavioral epigenetics, which suggests that the energy of psy-
cho-social relationships can be captured from methylation of the
genome and a subsequent change in gene expression. This could
explain why socially connected people live longer than do isolated
people.

So, we will potentially learn to alter our biological state by
changing our DNA or the expression of our DNA in the years to

come. How will we learn what to do? This is where embracing the science, partaking in online communities will come into play. We have become a quick fix society. We crave fast food and get rich quick schemes. But it is in the process of health that this is most evident. We want a pill or even an operation to fix our problems. When we are told that it may not work, we don't listen because we know someone that took the pill or had the operation and is doing better. Or worse, we saw an ad on the TV of someone who is doing better. The key will be to think for ourselves and to manage our own health.

There is a second component to epigenetics that involves memes. These are inheritable systems of beliefs that allow for meaningful changes in living that are "outside" of the genome as well. The way we are taught by our parents and the social norms that we are exposed to may have an influence on how our brains actually develop.

Again, online communities have the potential to intensify the effects of memes by democratizing our thought processes and facilitating their spread. Patients will dictate these processes while doctors will continue to be indispensable as partners in the process.

Adam might have focused less on having the surgeon "fix" his back and the insurance company trying to save money and more on how he was going to change his back, himself, with exercise. Rather than look for a quick fix, he could embrace the "slow fix."

Aesop said that the rabbit runs faster than the fox because the rabbit is running for its life while the fox is only running for its dinner. I would have urged Adam to play the part of the rabbit for just one purpose, to take control of his health.

In the long run, however the mindset of the rabbit's other nemesis, the turtle, should have been Adam's role model. While taking responsibility is vital and urgent, the actual process of acquiring health requires dedication, patience, and refection. It is adapting a "slow-fix" in a seductive world that promotes the "quick-fix."

CHAPTER 19

Internet Medicine

The last chapter gave you a glance into how narratives may transform the office visit of the future. The office visit will only be a small part of the narrative medicine of the future. The Internet will provide the necessary transparency and access to the narratives of both doctors and patients to allow them to become the essence of health acquisition. It will allow for the Me in Medicine to thrive.

In chapter 17, I suggested that the actionable medium of the Internet could not only improve health, but even alter disease. At this point in the book you must realize that "disease" is a somewhat arbitrary, organizational construct that arose to facilitate treatment and either assume cause for a set of symptoms or facilitate the business of medicine. The Internet will allow patients and doctors to describe a "set of symptoms" rather substitute a specific disease for this set of symptoms. More importantly, this "set of symptoms" will be further characterized as uniquely experienced by an individual patient. Getting away from traditional and static definitions of disease and creating new definitions for clusters of symptoms related to specific individuals will allow for more meaningful connections between the symptoms and potential treatments.

Do you remember the problem with Alexis's MRI report, which was limited by the interpretation and language of an individual radiologist? Similar to the idea of replacing disease with a "set of symptoms" is replacing the MRI report with a quantitative rendering of the data. Rather than talk about herniated discs versus bulging discs, the report will quantify the disc height, hydration, shape, and canal compromise. The report doesn't need a diagnosis at the end. The closest Alexis needed to get to diagnosis was a summation of her symptoms, physical limitations, MRI quantitative findings, and response to treatment.

One of the problems with back pain as a diagnosis or disease entity is that the words "back pain" may be an umbrella term for many different sets of symptoms. When we apply evidence-based medicine, we cannot currently come up with a predictive treatment for acute back pain. If we subdivide back pain into *sets of symptoms for a unique patient* and then apply evidence-based scrutiny, we may be able to come up with treatments with predictable efficacy.

If we withdraw from the importance of disease and MRI reports and allow our advanced computer capabilities to manage and track the complicated and unique symptoms and radiologic findings of our patients, our narratives will become essential in a world that appears less black and white. Our patient's capacity to alter their predicaments by communicating with similarly afflicted patients and experienced doctors will further bolster the power of the narrative.

When a patient comes to see me with a back problem I have already suggested that I need to find the right treatment not only for that particular condition, but for that particular patient with that particular problem. Our enhanced data stores will increasingly allow for that capability as more data becomes available and usable.

As patients participate by adding their own interpretation of their sets of symptoms and their response to treatments, the information available for evidence-based medicine will increase. In this way, patients will not only improve their health, they will alter the concepts of each disease or diagnosis. This is a provocative idea. It is similar to the concept of Wikipedia. Who would have thought that traditional experts would be replaced by a collective, dynamic, and shared expertise? Medicine will be similarly democratized and the concepts of disease and diagnosis will become more dynamic and collectively orchestrated.

The Internet provides the opportunity to form online communities that similarly have the potential to transform medicine. Traditionally, patients who come to their doctors with a known disease have been limited to the experience and advice of that doctor. Success in this model presupposes that the doctor has had access to all of the cutting-edge research, the most modern breakthroughs, or the many other forms of progress in treating a disease. This is, of course, not the case. Patients are an invaluable source of information and experience for one another. They are also a tremendous source of inspiration and willpower. The way that one individual deals with a problem is distinct from the way that another individual deals with the same problem. If the group is orchestrated properly, it can be a source of creativity and change as it provides not one approach but many.

Online communities will serve such a function in the future. In this setting, the doctors will be part of these communities as well. I believe that the doctors will hold a special place, but that will be an earned privilege and not an automatic one. This will force more subspecialization among doctors because a "jack of all trades" will no longer suffice in a democratized world where basic information is readily available. The doctor will also learn from his participation in these online communities.

There is big difference between simply experiencing something and experiencing something with the intention to share it—to edit and teach it. Patients must not only learn on the Internet, they must become part of its interactive medium. They must become an editor of its content.

Look what has happened to our evening news. We have been transitioned from being told what is important (traditional 6 o'clock news) to finding what we find important (niche Internet sites) and finally to writing our own news (sharing stories on Facebook or writing blogs). By sharing and writing, we will not just be learning and thinking better, we will be committing to and sharing our ideas. By trying to affect others we will be affecting change in ourselves. Writing has many benefits to patients. It allows for connection and rapid dissemination of ideas and treatments. David McCullough, the famous biographer, believes that writing is thinking. Writing well is clear thinking. That is why writing is so hard. But there is a benefit as the process of writing clarifies and potentiates the process of learning.

We need to think of medicine not as revolving around doctors and hospitals, but as part of our communities and social networks. Just as we have learned to share personal stories or interesting ideas on Facebook, we must use the power of communities and sharing to extend our health. We can share how many steps we have taken, the type of foods we have eaten, or the bad habits we have broken. The process of partaking in such relationships requires us to author our intents. It is in this authorship that we transition to being owners of our health.

As I stated for doctors, there is a great difference between learning and writing what one has learned. When patients convey what they have learned about health on a community blog site, the experience is transformative. They are not supposed to be doctors, but simply trying to be more like doctors. What a patient has to say will offer patients a different perspective.

If one pictures the Internet as a vast, accessible, and dynamic receptacle for health information, persuasion and influence will be paramount and need to be earned. We have already discussed how transparency of information makes empathy vital in our persuasion and influence. Aristotle suggested that persuasion consists of three modes: the ethos, the logos, and the pathos.

While *ethos* (reputation) and *logos* (ability) are important, *pathos* (the emotional aspect) reigns supreme in my opinion. It provides the framework for an optimal doctor-patient encounter. An emotional connection or passion between doctor and patient serves to facilitate communication, enhance trust, and allow the diagnosis and treatment to resonate with both doctor and patient. This is the most nuanced aspect of the encounter—whether in person or via the Internet. Again, both doctor and patient share this responsibility. I have learned not only the importance of *conveying* a genuine interest, but that I must also *have* an interest.

How do I create passion in my relationships with my patients? How do my patients become passionate about me? This is the point of this whole book. You can't act the part without being the part. Being the part requires deliberate and hard work with dedicated development of our character and the production of narratives through engagement and transparency. Listening carefully to the each other's narratives, sharing those narratives, and creating new, shared narratives is what the Me in Medicine is all about.

Bibliography

Anderson, Chris. *The Long Tail: Why the Future of Business Is Selling Less of More*. New York: Hyperion, 2008.

Brooks, David. *The Road to Character*. London: Allen Lane, 2015.

Carey, Nessa. *The Epigenetics Revolution: How Modern Biology Is Rewriting Our Understanding of Genetics, Disease, and Inheritance*. New York: Columbia University Press, 2013.

Carr, Nicholas G. *The Glass Cage: How Our Computers Are Changing Us*. New York: W.W. Norton, 2015.

Carr, Nicholas G. *The Shallows: What the Internet Is Doing to Our Brains*. New York: W.W. Norton, 2011.

Chabris, Christopher F., and Daniel J. Simons. *The Invisible Gorilla: How Our Intuitions Deceive Us*. Easton, PA: Harmony, 2011.

Connor, Stephen R., Bruce Pyenson, Kathryn Fitch, Carol Spence, and Kosuke Iwasaki. "Comparing Hospice and Nonhospice Patient Survival Among Patients Who Die Within a Three-Year Window." *Journal of Pain and Symptom Management* 33, no. 3 (March 2007), 238–246.

Csikszentmihalyi, Mihaly. *Flow: The Psychology of Optimal Experience*. New York: Harper and Row, 1990.

Gawande, Atul. *Being Mortal: Medicine and What Matters in the End*. New York: Metropolitan Books, Henry Holt and Company, 2014.

Gawande, Atul. "Overkill." *The New Yorker* 91, no. 12 (May 11, 2015), 42–55.

Gawande, Atul. "Tell Me Where It Hurts." *The New Yorker* 92, no. 46 (January 23, 2017), 36–-45.

Gilbert, Daniel Todd. *Stumbling on Happiness*. New York: A.A. Knopf, 2006.

Grant, Adam M. *Give and Take: Why Helping Others Drives Our Success*. New York: Viking, 201.

Groopman, Jerome E. *How Doctors Think*. Boston: Houghton Mifflin, 2008.

Groopman, Jerome, and Pamela Hartzband. *Your Medical Mind: How to Decide What Is Right for You*. New York: Penguin Press, 2011.

Hadler, Nortin M. *By the Bedside of the Patient: Lessons for the Twenty-First-Century Physician*. Chapel Hill: University of North Carolina Press, 2016.

Hadler, Nortin M. *The Citizen Patient: Reforming Health Care for the Sake of the Patient, Not the System*. Chapel Hill: University of North Carolina Press, 2013.

Hadler, Nortin M. *Stabbed in the Back: Confronting Back Pain in an Over-treated Society*. Chapel Hill: University of North Carolina Press, 2009.

Hadler, Nortin M. *Worried Sick: A Prescription for Health in an Overtreated Society*. Chapel Hill: University of North Carolina Press, 2008.

Hannan, Edward L., Dinesh Kumar, Michael Racz, Albert L. Siu, and Mark R. Chassin. "New York State's Cardiac Surgery Reporting System: Four Years Later." *The Annals of Thoracic Surgery* 58, no. 6 (December 1994), 1852–1857.

Lanza, Robert, Bob Berman, and Alan McKnight. *Biocentrism: How Life and Consciousness Are the Keys to Understanding the True Nature of the Universe*. Dallas: BenBella Books, 2010.

Lieberman, Matthew D. *Social: Why Our Brains Are Wired to Connect*. New York: Crown Publishers, 2013.

Mukherjee, Siddhartha. "The Same Different." *The New Yorker* 92, no. 12 (May 2, 2016), 24–30.

Mukherjee, Siddhartha, and Santino Fontana. *The Laws of Medicine: Field Notes from an Uncertain Science*. New York: TED Books, Simon & Schuster, 2015.

Newport, Cal. *Deep Work: Rules for Focused Success in a Distracted World*. New York: Grand Central Publishing, 2018.

Newport, Cal. *So Good They Can't Ignore You: Why Skills Trump Passion in the Quest for Work You Love*. New York: Business Plus, 2012.

Ofri, Danielle. *What Doctors Feel: How Emotions Affect the Practice of Medicine*. Boston: Beacon Press, 2014.

Pink, Daniel H. *To Sell Is Human: The Surprising Truth About Moving Others*. New York: Riverhead Books, 2012.

Prasad, Vinayak K., and Adam S. Cifu. *Ending Medical Reversal: Improving Outcomes, Saving Lives*. Baltimore: Johns Hopkins University Press, 2015.

Rhoades, Donna R., Kay F. McFarland, W. Holmes Finch, and Andrew O. Johnson. "Speaking and Interruptions During Primary Care Office Visits." *Family Medicine* 33, no. 7 (July 2001), 528–532.

Schulz, Kathryn. *Being Wrong: Adventures in the Margin of Error*. New York: Ecco, 201.

Specter, Michael. "The Power of Nothing." *The New Yorker* 87, no. 40 (December 12, 2011), 30–36.

Tetlock, Philip. *Superforecasting: The Art and Science of Prediction*. New York: Random House, 2016.

Wachter, Robert M. *The Digital Doctor: Hope, Hype, and Harm at the Dawn of Medicine's Computer Age*. New York: McGraw-Hill Education, 2015.

Wallach, Joel D., Ma Lan, and G. N. Schrauzer. *Epigenetics: The Death of the Genetic Theory of Disease Transmission*. New York: SelectBooks, 2014.

About the Author

Patrick Roth, M.D., is the Chairman of Neurosurgery at Hackensack University Medical Center and the director of its neurosurgical residency training program. Dr. Roth has practiced neurosurgery in New Jersey for the past twenty years. He has been a perennial recipient of Castle and Connolly "Top Doctors" and has been featured in *New York Magazine*'s "Best Doctors" and *New Jersey Magazine*'s "Top Doctors."

Dr. Roth has authored numerous articles on the spine and been a contributing author in many neurosurgical publications. He also authors a blog that focuses on patient empowerment and the art, versus the science, of being a physician. The blog shares with the reader the perspective of a surgeon "without a scalpel."

Dr. Roth lives in northern New Jersey with his wife, two children, and border collie. An avid athlete and tennis player, he has also competed in triathlons. His lifelong interest in fitness and diet has shaped his focus on minimally invasive and non-operative solutions to back pain.

NOTES